# Essential Oils Cross Reference Guide
# Cross Referencing Over 110 Oils, Properties & Uses

### By Chas R. Harrison

© Chas R. Harrison (2015). All rights reserved.

No part of this publication may be reproduced, stored in or introduced into a retrieval system, or transmitted in any form or by any means (electronic, mechanical, photocopying, recording, or otherwise) without the prior permission of the copyright owner. Distribution, scanning or uploading this book via the internet or via any other means without the permission of the copyright owner is illegal and punishable by law. I would ask that you purchase only authorized electronic editions and do not participate in or encourage electronic piracy of copyrighted materials. Small passages may be quoted for review purposes if credit is given to the copyright holder. Your respect for the author's rights is appreciated.

Harrison, Chas (2015) "Essential Oils Cross Reference Guide
Cross Referencing Over 110 Oils, Properties & Uses" Print Edition.

**DISCLAIMER:** The statements and/or information contained in this book have not been evaluated by the Food and Drug Administration. This book is to share our experiences and to help educate the reader only. It is not intended as a substitute for medical advice. This information is not intended to diagnose, treat, cure, or prevent any disease, illness or injury. The author shall not be held liable or responsible with respect to any loss, damage or injury caused or alleged to be caused directly or indirectly by the information contained in this book. As stated elsewhere, people suffering from any disease, illness, or injury should consult a qualified health care professional.

**WARNING:** Essential oils can react adversely with pharmaceutical medications. They can also cause skin irritation and be extremely caustic to the eyes. If you have an illness or a condition requiring medication, always consult your medical provider before using EOs. The use of EOs by children or pregnant women should also first be cleared by a properly licensed medical provider.

This book is **not intended to be a complete guide** on the use of essential oils; it is intended to be a handy cross reference between oils, their uses, best oils to blend with, and their properties. The information contained here has been gathered from numerous sources and has not been confirmed as to its accuracy. A list of those resources are at the end of the book. There are numerous studies and "proofs" throughout the net for those wishing to study these oils in further detail.

If you find this book helpful, please leave a QUICK REVIEW on Amazon. That would be greatly appreciated. You can also see my OTHER BOOKS there. You can visit my website at chasharrison.com to sign up for free offers on eBooks, audio books and print offers.

# TOC

| | |
|---|---|
| PROBLEM SEARCH A-B | 4 |
| PROBLEM SEARCH C-D | 8 |
| PROBLEM SEARCH E-G | 14 |
| PROBLEM SEARCH H-J | 17 |
| PROBLEM SEARCH K-M | 21 |
| PROBLEM SEARCH N-R | 24 |
| PROBLEM SEARCH S | 27 |
| PROBLEM SEARCH T-Z | 30 |
| OIL SEARCH A-B | 33 |
| OIL SEARCH C | 36 |
| OIL SEARCH D-G | 40 |
| OIL SEARCH H-L | 43 |
| OIL SEARCH M-P | 46 |
| OIL SEARCH R-Z | 50 |
| PROPERTY SEARCH A-A | 54 |
| PROPERTY SEARCH B-E | 59 |
| PROPERTY SEARCH F-M | 63 |
| PROPERTY SEARCH N-Z | 65 |
| APPLYING/USING ESSENTIAL OILS | 68 |
| BLENDING ESSENTIAL OILS | 71 |
| REFERENCES | 72 |

# Problem Search A-B

**ABDOMINAL CRAMPS:** blue cypress, calendula, cardamom, clove, cumin, fennel, ginger, lavender, lemon, nutmeg, oregano, patchouli, peppermint, Roman chamomile, spearmint, tarragon, wintergreen

**ACNE:** benzoin, bergamot, cajeput, camphor, cedarwood, clove, galbanum, geranium, goldenrod, helichrysum, juniper, lemon, litsea cubeba, lovage leaf, mandarin, myrtle, palmarosa, parsley seed, petitgrain, Roman chamomile, tansy, tea tree

**ALERTNESS:** basil, cinnamon, clary sage, cypress, fennel, frankincense, geranium, grapefruit, juniper, lavender, lemon, lemongrass, lime, marjoram, melissa, myrrh, orange, patchouli, peppermint, pine, Roman chamomile, rosemary, sandalwood, thyme, vetiver, white fir, wintergreen, ylang-ylang

**ALLERGIES:** basil, blue tansy, eucalyptus, fennel, frankincense, ginger, grapefruit, lavender, lemon, lemongrass, melaleuca, orange, oregano, patchouli, peppermint, Roman chamomile, sandalwood, white fur

**AMENORRHEA:** bay laurel, blue yarrow, Bulgarian rose, carrot seed, celery seed, chamomile, clary sage, dill seed, fennel, green yarrow, hops flower, hyssop, juniper berry, lemon balm, lovage leaf, marjoram, myrrh, parsley seed, rosemary, tarragon

**ANEMIA:** carrot seed, cinnamon, citrus oils, frankincense, ginger, grapefruit, lavender, lemon, peppermint, ylang-ylang

**ANGER:** allspice, angelica, balsam fir, basil, bergamot, cassia, catnip, cedarwood, cinnamon, clary sage, coriander, fennel, frankincense, German chamomile, grapefruit, hinoki, ho wood, hops, hyssop, juniper, lavandin, lavender, lemon balm, lemon, marjoram, neroli, orange, patchouli, peppermint, petitgrain, rose, sandalwood, spikenard, St. John's wort, valerian, vanilla, vetiver, ylang ylang

**ANOREXIA:** angelica, basil, bay, bergamot, black pepper, cardamom, carrot seed, chamomile, cilantro, cinnamon, cistus oils, clary sage, clove, coriander, cumin, dill, fennel, frankincense, ginger, grapefruit, hyssop, lavender, lemon, lemongrass, marjoram, nutmeg, oregano, palmarosa, patchouli, peppermint, Roman chamomile, rosemary, sage, spearmint, tarragon, thyme, vetiver

**ANXIETY:** basil, bergamot, cassia, cinnamon, clary sage, clove, coriander, fennel, frankincense, grapefruit, lavender, lemon, marjoram, orange, peppermint, Roman chamomile, ylang-ylang

**APPETITE/INCREASE :** bitter orange, black pepper, clove, fennel, ginger, grapefruit, mace, melaleuca

**ARTHRITIS:** allspice, basil, bay laurel, benzoin, black spruce, camphor, cardamom, cedarwood, celery seed, cilantro, cistus, clove, cypress, eucalyptus, geranium, ginger, helichrysum, Idaho blue spruce, juniper, lavender, lemongrass, mace, marjoram, oregano, parsley seed, peppermint, pimento, pine, Roman chamomile, rosemary, St. John's wort, tumeric, white fir, wintergreen

**ASTHMA:** balsam fir, bay laurel, benzoin, blue tansy, cajeput, celery seed, clary sage, clove, cypress, eucalyptus, frankincense, geranium, hinoki, lavender, lemon, marjoram, myrrh, orange, oregano, peppermint, Roman chamomile, rosemary, tangerine

**ATHLETE'S FOOT:** basil, blue cypress, cilantro, cypress, elemi, eucalyptus, geranium, grapefruit, lavender, lemongrass, manuka, melaleuca, myrrh, oregano, peppermint, pine, tea tree, thyme

**BACK PAIN:** basil, cassia, clary sage, cypress, eucalyptus, geranium, lavender, marjoram, oregano, peppermint, Roman chamomile, rosemary, sandalwood, thyme, wintergreen

**BACTERIAL INFECTION:** basil, cassia, cinnamon, clary sage, clove, cypress, eucalyptus, frankincense, geranium, grapefruit, helichrysum, lavender, lemon, lemongrass, melaleuca, oregano, peppermint, rosemary, tangerine, thyme

**BAD BREATH:** cardamom, clove, fennel, ginger, grapefruit, lemon, lemongrass, mace, orange, peppermint

**BED WETTING:** basil, cypress, frankincense, marjoram, melaleuca, sandalwood

**BLADDER INFECTION:** basil, bergamot, cinnamon, clove, cypress, eucalyptus, fennel, frankincense, lavender, lemon, lemongrass, lime, *marjoram, melaleuca, orange, oregano, peppermint, sandalwood, thyme*

**BLEEDING EXTERNALLY:** *geranium, helichrysum, lavender*

**BLISTERS:** *basil, clary sage, cypress, frankincense, lavender, melaleuca, peppermint*

**BLOATING:** *bay laurel, cubeba, davana, ginger, juniper, ledum, lemon, litsea, peppermint, rosemary, wintergreen*

**BLOOD CLEANSER:** *eucalyptus, ginger, lavender, lemon, lemongrass, marjoram, peppermint, rosemary, thyme*

**BLOOD PRESSURE/LOW:** *cinnamon, lemon, orange, peppermint, rosemary*

**BLOOD PRESSURE/HIGH:** *celery seed, clary sage, clove, grapefruit, lavender, lemon balm, lemon, lemongrass, marjoram, rose, tansy, wintergreen, ylang ylang*

**BOILS:** *bergamot, cistus, clary sage, frankincense, galbanum, German chamomile, lavender, lemon, lemongrass, melaleuca, myrrh, niaouli, Roman chamomile*

**BOWEL CLEANSE:** *basil, chamomile, citrus oils, fennel, ginger, lavender, lemon, marjoram, peppermint, rosemary*

**BREAST TENDERNESS:** *clary sage, cypress, fennel, geranium, helichrysum, lemongrass, vetiver*

**BROKEN BONES:** *basil, clove, cypress, eucalyptus, frankincense, helichrysum, lemongrass, marjoram, melaleuca, sandalwood, white fir, wintergreen*

**BRONCHITIS:** *allspice, anise seed, balsam fir, basil, bay laurel, benzoin, bergamot, cajeput, camphor, clary sage, clove, copaiba, cypress, elemi, eucalyptus, fir needle, frankincense, ginger, hinoki, Idaho blue spruce, lavender, lemon, marjoram, melaleuca, myrrh, peppermint, pine, Roman chamomile, rosemary, sandalwood, tagetes, thyme, white fir, wintergreen*

**BRUISES:** *fennel, geranium, helichrysum, lavender, lemongrass, marjoram, orange, parsley seed, peppermint, Roman chamomile, tansy, white fir, wintergreen*

**BULIMIA:** *angelica, basil, bay, bergamot, black pepper, cardamom, carrot seed, chamomile, cilantro, cinnamon, cistus oils, clary sage, clove, coriander, cumin, dill, fennel, frankincense, ginger, grapefruit, hyssop, lavender, lemon, lemongrass, marjoram, nutmeg, orange, oregano, palmarosa, patchouli, peppermint, Roman chamomile, rosemary, sage, spearmint, tarragon, thyme, vetiver*

**BUNIONS:** *basil, black pepper, clove, cypress, eucalyptus, frankincense, geranium, German chamomile, ginger, helichrysum, juniper, lavender, lemon, lemongrass, marjoram, peppermint, Roman chamomile, rose, rosemary, white fir, wintergreen*

**BURNS:** *basil, carrot seed, clove, cypress, fir needle, geranium, German chamomile, helichrysum, lavender, melaleuca, peppermint, Roman chamomile, St. John's wort, tea tree, wintergreen*

**BURSITIS:** *basil, bay laurel, birch, black pepper, cajeput, cinnamon, clary sage, clove, cypress, eucalyptus, fennel, frankincense, geranium, ginger, hyssop, juniper, lavender, lemon, lemongrass, marjoram, melaleuca, oregano, peppermint, Roman chamomile, rosemary, thyme, vetiver, white fir, wintergreen*

# Problem Search C-D

**CALLUSES:** basil, black pepper, cistus oils, clove, cypress, eucalyptus, frankincense, geranium, German chamomile, ginger, helichrysum, juniper, lavender, lemon, lemongrass, marjoram, oregano, peppermint, Roman chamomile, rose, rosemary, sandalwood, thyme, white fir, wintergreen

**CALMING:** allspice, basil, bergamot, cassia, cinnamon, clary sage, coriander, cypress, davana, fennel, frankincense, geranium, grapefruit, helichrysum, lavender, lemon, marjoram, melissa, myrrh, orange, patchouli, peppermint, petitgrain, Roman chamomile, rose, rosemary, sandalwood, vanilla, vetiver, white fir, wintergreen, ylang-ylang

**CANCER:** basil, cinnamon, clary sage, clove, frankincense, geranium, lavender, lemon, lemongrass, lime, myrrh, orange, rose, rosemary, sandalwood

**CANDIDA/THRUSH:** clove, eucalyptus, lavender, lemon, lemongrass, melaleuca, oregano, peppermint, rosemary, thyme

**CANKER SORES:** cilantro, lavender, lemon, melaleuca, myrrh, orange, oregano, Roman chamomile

**CARPAL TUNNEL:** basil, cinnamon, clove, cypress, eucalyptus, frankincense, geranium, ginger, helichrysum, lavender, lemon, lemongrass, marjoram, peppermint, Roman chamomile, rosemary, thyme, white fir, wintergreen

**CARTILAGE:** basil, birch, cypress, helichrysum, lavender, lemongrass, marjoram, peppermint, rosemary, thyme, vetiver, white fir

**CATARACTS: DO NOT USE OILS IN EYES!!!** cassia, clove, cypress, eucalyptus, lavender, lemongrass, peppermint

**CATARRH:** camphor, cedarwood, cypress, eucalyptus, frankincense, ginger, helichrysum, manuka, myrrh, primrose, rosemary

**CELLULITE:** *basil, cypress, fennel, geranium, grapefruit, juniper, lavender, lemon, lime, orange, oregano, parsley seed, rosemary, tangerine*

**CHAPPED LIPS:** *chamomile, frankincense, geranium, lavender, lemon, melaleuca, neroli, rose, sandalwood, ylang-ylang*

**CHARLEY HORSE:** *basil, clary sage, clove, cypress, grapefruit, lemongrass, marjoram, peppermint, Roman chamomile, rosemary, thyme, vetiver*

**CHILLS:** *basil, bergamot, black pepper, cassia, clove, eucalyptus, fir needle, frankincense, ginger, lavender, lemon, melaleuca, white fir*

**CHOLERA:** *cajeput, clove, rosemary*

**CHOLESTEROL/HIGH/PLAQUE:** *basil, cilantro, cinnamon, clary sage, cypress, frankincense, geranium, ginger, grapefruit, helichrysum, lavender, lemon, lemongrass, marjoram, melissa, orange, peppermint, rosemary, sandalwood, thyme, ylang-ylang*

**CIRCULATION:** *basil, Bay West Indies, benzoin, bergamot, black pepper, cilantro, cinnamon, cistus, clary sage, clove, cypress, eucalyptus, frankincense, galbanum, ginger, grapefruit, lavender, lemon, mace, marjoram, melaleuca, myrrh, nutmeg, orange, oregano, parsley seed, peppermint, pimento, Roman chamomile, rose, rosemary, sandalwood, tangerine, thyme, white fir, wintergreen*

**COLD SORES:** *basil, bergamot, blue cypress, cilantro, eucalyptus, geranium, lavender, lemon, manuka, melaleuca, myrrh, orange, oregano, Roman chamomile*

**COLDS:** *anise seed, balsam fir, basil, bay laurel, Bay West Indies, benzoin, black pepper, cajeput, camphor, cassia, cilantro, cinnamon, cistus, cubeba, cypress, eucalyptus, forado azil, frankincense, ginger, grapefruit, jasmine, ledum, lemon. lemongrass, lime, litsea, marjoram, melaleuca, oregano, peppermint, rosemary, tea tree, thyme*

**COLIC:** *bergamot, cajeput, cardamom, carrot seed, cilantro, fennel, ginger, marjoram, melissa, mountain savory, orange, peppermint, Roman chamomile, rosemary, ylang-ylang*

**COLITIS:** clove, frankincense, geranium, ginger, helichrysum, lemon, neroli, oregano, peppermint, rosemary, thyme

**COMPLEXION DRY:** (see dry skin) cedarwood, clary sage, frankincense, geranium, jasmine, lavender, lemon, myrtle, patchouli, Roman chamomile, rose, rosewood, sandalwood, ylang-ylang

**COMPLEXION OILY:** (see oily skin) bergamot, clary sage, cypress, frankincense, geranium, helichrysum, lavender, lemon, lemongrass, marjoram, orange, patchouli, peppermint, Roman chamomile, rosemary, sandalwood, tea tree, ylang-ylang

**CONCUSSION:** cilantro, clary sage, cypress, frankincense, geranium, helichrysum, lemon, lemongrass, orange, peppermint

**CONGESTION:** basil, bergamot, cedarwood, cinnamon, clary sage, clove, cypress, elemi, eucalyptus, frankincense, ginger, hinoki, lavender, ledum, lemon, marjoram, melaleuca, myrrh, myrtle, orange, oregano, peppermint, Roman chamomile, rosemary, sandalwood, tagetes, thyme, white fir, wintergreen

**CONSTIPATION:** carrot seed, copaiba, dill, fennel, ginger, lemon, mace, marjoram, orange, peppermint, rose, rosemary, sandalwood, tangerine, yarrow

**CORNS:** basil, cassia, clove, cypress, eucalyptus, grapefruit, helichrysum, lemon, myrrh, orange, oregano, peppermint, Roman chamomile, vetiver

**COUGH:** allspice, anise seed, balsam fir, basil, benzoin, bergamot, camphor, cardamom, cinnamon, cistus, clary sage, clove, cypress, dorado azil, elemi, eucalyptus, fir needle frankincense, ginger hinoki, ginger, jasmine, lavender, ledum, lemon, lemongrass, marjoram, melaleuca, myrrh, myrtle, orange, oregano, peppermint, pimento, Roman chamomile, rosemary, sandalwood, tagetes, thyme, white fir, wintergreen

**CRADLE CAP:** geranium, lavender, lemon, melaleuca, tea tree

**CRAMPS/MUSCLE:** basil, birch, catnip, clary sage, coriander, cypress, galbanum, ginger, helichrysum, hops, lavender, lemongrass, marjoram, mountain savory, peppermint, Roman chamomile, rosemary, thyme, tumeric, vetiver, white fir, white fir,    wintergreen, yarrow

**CROUP:** *clove, cypress, eucalyptus, frankincense, hyssop, lavender, lemon, marjoram, melaleuca, oregano, peppermint, ravensara, rosemary, sandalwood, thyme*

**CUTS/WOUNDS:** *basil, cassia, cinnamon, clary sage, clove, cypress, elemi, eucalyptus, frankincense, galbanum, geranium, grapefruit, helichrysum, Idaho blue spruce, lavender, lemon, lemongrass, marjoram, melaleuca, oregano, peppermint, pimento, Roman chamomile, rosemary, St. John's wort, tangerine, thyme, yarrow*

**CYSTITIS:** *basil, bergamot, cajeput, cassia, cedarwood, celery seed, cinnamon, clove, cypress, elemi, eucalyptus, fennel, frankincense, German chamomile, juniper, lavender, lavender, lemon, melaleuca, niaouli, oregano, palmarosa, parsley seed, pine, rosemary, rosewood, sage, sandalwood, tea tree, thyme*

**DANDRUFF:** *basil, Bay West Indies, cedarwood, cypress, geranium, juniper, lavender, manuka, melaleuca, pine, rosemary, sage, tangerine, thyme, wintergreen*

**DARK SPOTS:** *carrot seed, cypress, frankincense, geranium, grapefruit, helichrysum, lavender, lemon, mandarin, myrtle oregano, myrtle, neroli, patchouli, peppermint, Roman chamomile, sandalwood, tea tree, ylang-ylang*

**DECONGESTANT:** *amyris, basil, bergamot, cinnamon, clary sage, clove, cypress, eucalyptus, frankincense, ginger, hyssop, Idaho blue spruce, lavender, lemon, marjoram, melaleuca, myrrh, orange, oregano, patchouli, peppermint, Roman chamomile, rosemary, sandalwood, thyme, white fir, wintergreen*

**DENTAL ABSCESSES/INFECTIONS:** *basil, Bay West Indies, benzoin, clove, cornmint, frankincense, helichrysum, lemon, melaleuca, orange, Roman chamomile, wintergreen*

**DEODORANT:** *bergamot, clary sage, frankincense, geranium, lavender, lemon, lemongrass, melaleuca, orange, patchouli, peppermint, rosemary, sandalwood, tea tree, thyme, wintergreen*

**DEPRESSION:** *allspice, basil, benzoin, bergamot, birch, camphor, cassia, cinnamon, clary sage, clove, cypress, davana, fennel, frankincense, grapefruit, ho wood, jasmine, lavandin, lavender, lemon* balm, lemon, lime, marjoram, Melissa, melissa, neroli, orange, patchouli, peppermint, petitgrain, pine, Roman chamomile, rose, rosewood, sandalwood, thyme, valerian, vanilla, ylang ylang

**DERMATITIS:** bergamot, carrot seed, cistus, cypress, frankincense, geranium, German chamomile, helichrysum, juniper, lemon, lovage leaf, marjoram, melaleuca, orange, palmarosa, Roman chamomile, rosemary, tansy, thyme

**DETOX:** cassia, catnip, cilantro, clove, coriander, cypress, helichrysum, juniper, lemon, lemongrass, melaleuca, parsley seed, pine, rosemary, tangerine, thyme

**DIABETES:** basil, cassia, cinnamon, clary sage, clove, coriander, cypress, davana, dill, eucalyptus, frankincense, geranium, grapefruit, helichrysum, juniper, juniper., lavender, lemon, marjoram, peppermint, pine, thyme, vetiver, ylang-ylang

**DIAPER RASH:** calendula, chamomile, frankincense, lavender, melaleuca, Roman chamomile

**DIARRHEA:** Bay West Indies, black pepper, carrot seed, cilantro, copaiba, cypress, eucalyptus, geranium, ginger, lavender, melaleuca, mountain savory, myrrh, neroli, orange, peppermint, sandalwood, tangerine

**DIGESTION PROBLEMS:** allspice, bay laurel, black pepper, cajeput, celery seed, cilantro, cinnamon, davana, dill, fennel, ginger, juniper, lemongrass, marjoram, melaleuca, mountain savory, neroli, oregano, parsley seed, peppermint, spearmint, tangerine, tarragon, tumeric

**DIURETIC:** cypress, fennel, grapefruit, lavender, lemon, lemongrass, marjoram, orange, oregano, rosemary

**DIVERTICULITIS:** chamomile, cinnamon, clove, ginger, lavender, lemon, melaleuca, peppermint, ravensara, rosemary

**DRY SKIN:** (see skin health) blue cypress, carrot seed, cedarwood, cistus, elemi, geranium, German chamomile, jasmine, juniper, lemon balm, lovage leaf, Roman chamomile, sandalwood

**DYSENTERY:** basil, cinnamon, clove, coriander, cypress, dill, eucalyptus, fennel, frankincense, geranium, ginger, lemon, lemongrass, *melaleuca, melissa, mountain savory, myrrh, myrtle, orange, oregano, peppermint, Roman chamomile, rosemary, sandalwood, tea tree, thyme*

# Problem Search E-G

**EARACHE: DO NOT PUT DIRECTLY INTO EARS!!!** *basil, calendula, eucalyptus, helichrysum, lavender, lemon, male rose, marjoram, melaleuca, parsley seed, peppermint, rosemary, tea tree, thyme, wintergreen*

**ECZEMA:** *benzoin, bergamot, blue cypress, carrot seed, cedarwood, cistus, geranium, German chamomile, helichrysum, jasmine, juniper, lavender, lemon balm, lovage leaf, melaleuca, Roman chamomile, rosemary, sandalwood, thyme*

**EDEMA:** *bay laurel, carrot seed, cypress, fennel, geranium, grapefruit, grapefruit, juniper, lavender, lemon, lemongrass, lovage leaf, rosemary*

**ENERGY:** *basil, cilantro, eucalyptus, grapefruit, lavender, lemon, lemongrass, orange, peppermint, rosemary, sandalwood, tangerine, thyme, white fir*

**ESTROGEN:** *basil, clary sage, coriander, cypress, fennel, frankincense, geranium, German chamomile, grapefruit, lavender, lemon, oregano, tarragon, tea tree, thyme, ylang-ylang*

**EYES: DO NOT PUT DIRECTLY INTO EYES!!!** *cypress, eucalyptus, fennel, frankincense, lavender, lemon, lemongrass, melaleuca, peppermint, sandalwood*

**FAINTING:** *basil, black pepper, cedarwood, cilantro, cinnamon, frankincense, ginger, lavender, melissa, neroli, orange, oregano, patchouli, peppermint, Roman chamomile, rosemary*

**FAT/WEIGHT REDUCERS:** (see weight loss) *bergamot, blue tansy, cinnamon leaf, citruses, cypress, fennel, geranium, grapefruit, juniper, lavender, lemon, lemongrass, lime, orange, patchouli, peppermint, petitgrain, rosemary, sandalwood, tangerine, thyme, ylang-ylang*

**FATIGUE:** *angelica, basil, bergamot, cilantro, cistus oils, eucalyptus, fennel, frankincense, grapefruit, lavender, lemon, lemongrass, orange, peppermint, pine, rosemary, sandalwood, thyme, white fir*

**FEAR:** *basil, bergamot, cassia, cinnamon, clary sage, coriander, cypress, fennel, frankincense, geranium, grapefruit, helichrysum, lavender, lemon, marjoram, melissa, myrrh, orange, patchouli, peppermint, Roman chamomile, rose, sandalwood, white fir, wintergreen, vetiver, ylang ylang*

**FEVER:** *basil, bergamot, black pepper, cajeput, clove, cypress, eucalyptus, fir needle, frankincense, ginger, lavender, ledum, lemon, lime, melaleuca, niaouli, parsley seed, peppermint, white fir*

**FLATULENCE:** (see gas) *anise seed, basil, bergamot, cardamom, cilantro, cornmint, cypress, eucalyptus, fennel, geranium, ginger, lavender, melaleuca, myrrh, orange, peppermint, rosemary, sandalwood*

**FLU COLD:** *basil, bergamot, cinnamon, clary, clove, cypress, eucalyptus, frankincense, ginger, lavender, lemon, marjoram, melaleuca, myrrh, orange, oregano, peppermint, Roman chamomile, rosemary, sage, sandalwood, thyme, white fir, wintergreen*

**FLU STOMACH:** *anise seed, balsam fir, bay laurel, Bay West Indies, black pepper, camphor, cilantro, cinnamon, cistus, eucalyptus, ginger, ledum, lime, tea tree*

**FLUID RETENTION:** *cypress, geranium, grapefruit, juniper, lemon, lemongrass, marjoram, orange, parsley seed, rosemary, tangerine*

**FOOT ODOR:** (see deodorant) *citrus oils, melaleuca*

**FUNGAL INFECTION/CANDIDA:** *black pepper, cilantro, cinnamon, clove, eucalyptus, geranium, lavender, lemon, lemongrass, mandarin, manuka, melaleuca, myrrh, oregano, patchouli, peppermint, rosemary, tea tree, thyme, thyme*

**GALLBLADDER:** *carrot seed, geranium, helichrysum, lavender, lemon, peppermint, rose, rosemary, wintergreen*

**GALLSTONES:** *carrot seed, geranium, helichrysum, lavender, lemon peppermint ,rose, rosemary, wintergreen*

**GANGRENE:** *basil, geranium, grapefruit, helichrysum, lavender, lemon, lemongrass, marjoram, melaleuca, oregano, peppermint, rosemary, thyme*

**GAS:** (also see flatulence) *bay laurel, davana, dill, fennel*

**GERD/REFLUX:** *allspice, bay laurel, black pepper, cajeput, celery seed, cilantro, cinnamon, davana, dill, fennel, ginger, juniper, lemongrass, marjoram, melaleuca, mountain savory, neroli, oregano, parsley seed, peppermint, spearmint, tangerine, tangerine, tarragon, tumeric*

**GINGIVITIS:** *myrrh, helichrysum, melaleuca, orange, Roman chamomile, rose*

**GOUT:** *angelica, basil, cajeput, carrot seed, celery seed, cinnamon, clove, cypress, eucalyptus, frankincense, geranium, ginger, helichrysum, juniper, lavender, lemon, lemongrass, marjoram, nutmeg, peppermint, Roman chamomile, rosemary, tansy, thyme, white fir, wintergreen*

**GRIEF:** *basil, bergamot, cinnamon, clary sage, clove, cypress, fennel, frankincense, grapefruit, lavender, lemon, lime, marjoram, melissa, orange, peppermint, Roman chamomile, rose, sandalwood, ylang-ylang,*

**GROWING PAINS:** *basil, cypress, lavender, marjoram, orange, peppermint, sandalwood, white fir, wintergreen*

**GUMS:** *basil, clove, fennel, frankincense, ginger, helichrysum, melaleuca, myrrh, orange, Roman chamomile, rose*

# Problem Search H-J

**HAIR, DRY:** *geranium, lavender, rosemary, sandalwood, wintergreen*

**HAIR, OILY:** *basil, cypress, lemon, melaleuca, rosemary, thyme*

**HAIR LOSS:** *Bay West Indies, cedarwood, clary sage, cypress, grapefruit, lavender, lemon, marjoram, peppermint, Roman chamomile, rosemary, thyme, vetiver, ylang ylang*

**HANGOVER:** *cilantro, grapefruit, lavender, lemon, orange, peppermint, rosemary, sandalwood*

**HAY FEVER:** (see allergies) *cilantro, cypress, eucalyptus, lavender, peppermint, Roman chamomile, rose, vetiver*

**HEADACHE:** *basil, cajeput, cardamom, cilantro, clary sage, clove, cypress, eucalyptus, fennel, frankincense, German chamomile, grapefruit, lavandin, lavender, lemon balm, lemon, lemongrass, lime, marjoram, melaleuca, melissa, myrrh, orange, oregano, patchouli, peppermint, pimento, Roman chamomile, rosemary, sandalwood, spikenard, St. John's wort, vetiver, white fir, wintergreen, ylang-ylang*

**HEARING LOSS: DO NOT PUT DIRECTLY INTO EARS:** *almond, basil, cilantro, cypress, eucalyptus, fennel, geranium, helichrysum, juniper, lavender, marjoram, Roman chamomile, rosemary, tea tree, white fir*

**HEART HEALTH:** (see also circulation and blood cleanser) *celery seed, lavender, palmarosa, tansy, ylang ylang*

**HEART PALPITATIONS:** *basil, camphor, clary sage, cypress, frankincense, geranium, ginger, grapefruit, helichrysum, lavender, lemon, marjoram, melissa, neroli, orange, peppermint, pine, rosemary, sandalwood, thyme, vetiver, ylang-ylang*

**HEARTBURN:** *allspice, black pepper, cardamom, cilantro, cornmint, frankincense, ginger, grapefruit, hops, hyssop, lavender, lemon, mountain savory, myrrh, orange, peppermint, thyme, white fir, wintergreen*

**HEATSTROKE:** *clary sage, cypress, eucalyptus, lavender, lemon, lime, melaleuca, orange, peppermint, Roman chamomile, tangerine*

**HEMORRHOIDS:** *cistus, clary sage, copaiba, cypress, fir needle, frankincense, geranium, helichrysum, myrrh, parsley seed, peppermint, sandalwood, St. John's wort, white fir, wintergreen, yarrow*

**HEPATITIS:** *basil, cinnamon, cypress, eucalyptus, frankincense, melaleuca, myrrh, oregano, peppermint, Roman chamomile, rosemary, thyme*

**HERNIA:** *basil, cypress, fennel, geranium, ginger, lavender, lemon, melaleuca, rosemary*

**HERPES SIMPLEX:** *bergamot, clove, cypress, eucalyptus, geranium, helichrysum, lavender, lemon, melaleuca, oregano, peppermint, rose*

**HICCUPS:** *dill, fennel, lemon, orange, peppermint, sandalwood, tarragon*

**HIVES:** (see rash) *basil, cypress, lavender, melaleuca, peppermint, Roman chamomile*

**HOARSENESS:** (see laryngitis) *jasmine*

**HORMONE BALANCE:** *basil, cinnamon, clary sage, clove, cypress, Cypress, davana, fennel, frankincense, geranium, grapefruit, lavender, melissa, myrtle, orange, Roman chamomile, rose, rosemary, sage, thyme, ylang-ylang*

**HOT FLASHES:** *clary sage, melaleuca, peppermint*

**HYPOGLYCEMIA:** (see diabetes) *basil, cassia, cinnamon, clary sage, clove, coriander, cypress, davana, dill, eucalyptus, frankincense, geranium, grapefruit, helichrysum, juniper, lavender, lemon, marjoram, peppermint, pine, thyme, vetiver, ylang-ylang*

**HYPERTHYROID:** *lemongrass, myrrh*

**HYPOTHYROID:** *clove, lemongrass, peppermint*

**IMMUNOSTIMULANT:** *cistus, lavender, lemon, lime, marjoram, melaleuca, orange, oregano, peppermint, ravensara, tansy*

**IMPOTENCE:** *basil, bergamot, cilantro, clary sage, clove, ginger, goldenrod, jasmine, lemon, nutmeg, rose, sandalwood, thyme*

**INDIGESTION:** *allspice, black pepper, cardamom, cilantro, cornmint, frankincense, ginger, grapefruit, hops, hyssop, lavender, lemon, mountain savory, myrrh, orange, peppermint, thyme, white fir, wintergreen*

**INFECTION:** *balsam fir, basil, bay laurel, bergamot, blue cypress, camphor, cassia, cilantro, cinnamon, clary sage, clove, cypress, eucalyptus, frankincense, geranium, grapefruit, helichrysum, hyssop, Idaho blue spruce, lavender, lemon myrtle, lemon, lemongrass, lime, marjoram, melaleuca, myrrh, oregano, peppermint, ravensara, rosemary, tea tree, thyme*

**INFERTILITY/MALE:** *basil, clary sage, thyme*

**INFLAMMATION:** *bergamot, blue tansy, camphor, cinnamon, clary sage, eucalyptus, galbanum, hyssop, lavandin, lavender, lemongrass, myrrh, nutmeg, oregano, peppermint, Roman chamomile, tumeric, wintergreen*

**INSECT BITES:** *basil, bergamot, cajeput, cinnamon, copaiba, cypress, eucalyptus, helichrysum, lavender, lemon, lemongrass, melaleuca, niaouli, patchouli, peppermint, Roman chamomile, sage, thyme*

**INSECT REPELLANT:** *basil, blue cypress, camphor, catnip, citronella, cubeba, lavender, lemon balm, lemongrass, litsea, melaleuca, palo santo, tagetes, tansy*

**INSECT STINGS:** *basil, bergamot, cajeput, cinnamon, copaiba, cypress, helichrysum, lavender, lemon, lemongrass, melaleuca, niaouli, patchouli, peppermint, Roman chamomile, sage, thyme*

**INSOMNIA:** *basil, bergamot, catnip, clary sage, cypress, fennel, frankincense, German chamomile, hops, jasmine, juniper, lavender, lemon balm, lemon, mandarin, marjoram, melissa, myrrh, neroli, orange, peppermint, petitgrain, Roman chamomile, rosemary, sandalwood, spikenard, valerian, vanilla, vetiver, white fir, ylang-ylang*

**ITCHING:** *basil, cedarwood, cypress, lavender, lemongrass, manuka, patchouli, peppermint, Roman chamomile, rosemary, sandalwood*

**JAUNDICE:** *geranium, lemon, rosemary*

**JOINT RELIEF/HEALTH:** *basil, cypress, helichrysum, lavender, lemongrass, marjoram, peppermint, rosemary, thyme, vetiver, white fir, wintergreen*

# Problem Search K-M

**KIDNEY INFECTION/CLEANSE:** *celery seed, clary sage, eucalyptus, geranium, grapefruit, ledum, lemon, lemongrass, rosemary, spruce, tansy, thyme*

**LACTOSE INTOLERANCE:** *lemon, lemongrass*

**LARYNGITIS:** *cajeput, frankincense, ginger, jasmine, lavender, ledum, lemon, niaouli, sandalwood, thyme*

**LICE:** *eucalyptus, geranium, lavender, lemon, lemongrass, manuka, melaleuca, rosemary*

**LIGAMENT INJURIES:** *basil, birch, cypress, helichrysum, lavender, lemongrass, marjoram, peppermint, rosemary, thyme, vetiver, white fir, wintergreen*

**LIPS:** *lavender, lemon, melaleuca, rose*

**LIVER CLEANSE/REPAIR:** *bay laurel, blue tansy, carrot seed, clove, cypress, frankincense, geranium, German chamomile, goldenrod, grapefruit, helichrysum, ledum, lemon, myrtle, parsley seed, Roman chamomile, rose*

**LUNGS:** (see respiratory) *cypress, eucalyptus, frankincense, melaleuca, sandalwood*

**LYMPH SYSTEM/GLANDS:** *basil, bergamot, blue tansy, cinnamon, clary sage, clove, cypress, eucalyptus, frankincense, ginger, grapefruit, lavender, lemon, marjoram, melaleuca, myrrh, orange, oregano, peppermint, Roman chamomile, rosemary, sandalwood, tangerine, thyme, white fir, wintergreen*

**MALARIA:** *basil, cassia, cinnamon, clary sage, clove, cypress, eucalyptus, frankincense, geranium, grapefruit, helichrysum, lavender, lemon, lemongrass, marjoram, melaleuca, oregano, peppermint, rosemary, thyme*

**MEASLES:** *eucalyptus, lavender, melaleuca*

**MELANOMA:**  *bergamot, frankincense, grapefruit, lemon, lime, orange, sandalwood, tangerine*

**MEMORY:**  *basil, bergamot, cilantro, clary sage, clove, cypress, frankincense, ginger, grapefruit, lavender, lemongrass, peppermint, rosemary*

**MENOPAUSE:**  *basil, clary sage, cypress, fennel, galbanum, geranium, German chamomile, jasmine, lavender, melissa, orange, Roman chamomile, rosemary, sage, thyme, ylang-ylang*

**MENSTRUAL CRAMPING:**  *basil, cistus, clary sage, clove, cypress, geranium, German chamomile, grapefruit, jasmine, juniper, lemongrass, lovage leaf, marjoram, myrrh, nutmeg, parsley seed, peppermint, Roman chamomile, rose, rosemary, sage, tarragon, thyme, vetiver, yarrow*

**MENTAL ALERTNESS:**  (see alertness) *basil, cardamom, coriander, hyssop, jasmine, pine, rosemary, spearmint*

**METABOLISM:**  *clove, oregano*

**MOLES:**  *geranium, frankincense, lavender, oregano, sandalwood*

**MOLLUSCUM CONTAGIOSUM:**  *lemon, myrtle, tea tree*

**MONONUCLEOSIS:**  *basil, bergamot, cinnamon, clary sage, clove, cypress, eucalyptus, frankincense, ginger, lavender, lemon, marjoram, melaleuca, myrrh, orange, oregano, peppermint, Roman chamomile, rosemary, sandalwood, thyme, white fir, wintergreen*

**MORNING SICKNESS:**  (see nausea) *ginger, orange, peppermint*

**MOTION SICKNESS:**  (see nausea) *ginger, orange, peppermint, vetiver*

**MRSA:**  (see bacterial infections) *cinnamon, clove, eucalyptus, geranium, grapefruit, lavender, lemon, lemongrass, melaleuca, orange, oregano, peppermint, thyme*

**MUMPS:**  (see viruses) *basil, cypress, eucalyptus, lavender, lemon, melaleuca, peppermint*

**MUSCLE ACHES/PAIN:** *allspice, anise see, balsam fir, basil, Bay West Indies, benzoin, birch, black pepper, black spruce, blue cypress, blue tansy, camphor, cilantro, cinnamon, cypress, elemi, galbanum, ginger, grapefruit, helichrysum, jasmine, lavender, lemongrass, mace, marjoram, nutmeg, oregano, peppermint, pimento, pine, rosemary, St. John's wort, thyme, tumeric, vetiver, white fir, wintergreen*

**MUSCLE RELAXANT:** (see muscle aches/pains) *amyris, angelica, catnip*

**MUSCLE SPASM:** (see muscle aches/pains) *basil, clary sage, cypress, lavender, marjoram, peppermint, petitgrain, Roman chamomile*

# Problem Search N-R

**NAIL INFECTIONS/FUNGAL:** (see fungal infections) *cypress, eucalyptus, frankincense, grapefruit, lavender, lemon, melaleuca, myrrh, oregano, rosemary, thyme*

**NAILS BRITTLE/WEAK:** *almond, balsam fir, flax seed, frankincense, lemon, myrrh, vetiver, white fir, wintergreen*

**NAUSEA:** *allspice, black pepper, cajeput, cardamom, cilantro, clove, cornmint, fennel, ginger, lavender, mountain savory, orange, peppermint, tumeric*

**NERVOUSNESS:** *allspice, basil, bergamot, catnip, cedarwood, cinnamon, cistus, clary sage, cypress, elemi, fennel, frankincense, geranium, German chamomile, ginger, goldenrod, grapefruit, hinoki, ho wood, hops, jasmine, jasmine, juniper, lavandin, lavender, lemon, lime, marjoram, melissa, myrrh, neroli, orange, patchouli, peppermint, petitgrain, Roman chamomile, rose, rosemary, sandalwood, spikenard, St. John's wort, valerian, vanilla, vetiver, white fir, ylang-ylang*

**NEUROPATHY/NEURALGIA:** (see pain, inflammation) *allspice, Bay West Indies*

**NIGHT SWEATS:** *bergamot, carrot seed, cedarwood, clary sage, fennel, geranium, lavender, palmarosa, peppermint, primrose, sage, ylang-ylang*

**NOSE BLEED:** *cypress, helichrysum, frankincense, lavender, lemon*

**OCD/OBSESSIVE COMPULSIVE DISORDER:** (see calming) *carrot seed, cedarwood, fennel, juniper, lavender, lemon, litsea cubeba, mandarin, myrtle*

**OILY SKIN:** *Bay West Indies, petitgrain*

**OVARIAN PAIN:** (see pain) *basil, cilantro, clary sage, cypress, geranium, rosemary*

**PAIN:** *balsam fir, basil, black pepper, blue tansy, cajeput, chamomile, clary sage, clove, cypress, eucalyptus, frankincense, ginger, helichrysum, hops, juniper, lavender, marjoram, myrrh, oregano, peppermint, Roman chamomile, rosemary, sandalwood, thyme, vetiver, white fir, wintergreen, yarrow*

**PANCREAS:** *basil, cinnamon, coriander, cypress, cypress, fennel, frankincense, geranium, helichrysum, lemon, marjoram, rosemary, vetiver*

**PANIC ATTACK:** *allspice, basil, bergamot, cassia, cinnamon, clary sage, coriander, cypress, davana, fennel, frankincense, geranium, grapefruit, helichrysum, lavender, lemon, marjoram, melissa, myrrh, orange, patchouli, peppermint, petitgrain, Roman chamomile, rose, rosemary, sandalwood, valerian, vanilla, vetiver, white fir, wintergreen, ylang-ylang*

**PARASITES:** *clove, davana, fir needle, hyssop, lemon, melaleuca, mountain savory, niaouli, oregano, Roman chamomile, tarragon, thyme*

**PIMPLES/ACNE:** *clary sage, clove, eucalyptus, frankincense, geranium, lavender, lemon, lemongrass, marjoram, melaleuca, orange, rosemary, sandalwood, thyme, vetiver*

**PMS:** *basil, bergamot, clary sage, clove, cypress, fennel, frankincense, galbanum, geranium, grapefruit, jasmine, lavender, lemon, lemongrass, marjoram, melaleuca, peppermint, Roman chamomile, rosemary, tarragon, thyme, vetiver, wintergreen*

**PNEUMONIA:** *basil, bergamot, cinnamon, clary sage, clove, cypress, eucalyptus, frankincense, ginger, lavender, lemon, marjoram, melaleuca, myrrh, oregano, peppermint, Roman chamomile, rosemary, sandalwood, thyme, white fir, wintergreen*

**PROSTATE:** *cilantro, clary sage, clove, cypress, fennel, frankincense, geranium, helichrysum, lavender, myrrh, myrtle, oregano, peppermint, rosemary, thyme*

**PSORIASIS:** *angelica, benzoin, bergamot, cajeput, carrot seed, frankincense, German chamomile, helichrysum, juniper, lavender, melaleuca, Roman chamomile, rosemary, thyme*

**RASH:**  basil, benzoin, blue cypress, cajeput, carrot seed, cilantro, cypress, elemi, German chamomile, lavender, melaleuca, palmarosa, peppermint, Roman chamomile, spikenard

**REFLUX/GERD:**  allspice, bay laurel, black pepper, cajeput, celery seed, cilantro, cinnamon, davana, dill, fennel, ginger, juniper, lemongrass, marjoram, melaleuca, mountain savory, neroli, oregano, parsley seed, peppermint, spearmint, tangerine, tarragon, tumeric

**RESPIRATORY:**  (see bronchitis and asthma)  anise seed, cypress, dorado azil, Douglas fir, elemi, eucalyptus, frankincense, hyssop, melaleuca, melissa, sandalwood, spruce

**RHEUMATISM:**  allspice, balsam fir, basil, bay laurel, Bay West Indies, benzoin, black pepper, black spruce, cajeput, camphor, carrot seed, cedarwood, celery seed, cilantro, cinnamon, clove, cypress, eucalyptus, frankincense, geranium, ginger, helichrysum, Idaho blue spruce, lavender, lemon, lemongrass, marjoram, oregano, peppermint, pimento, pine, Roman chamomile, rosemary, thyme, tumeric, white fir, wintergreen

**RINGWORM:**  (see fungal infections)  blue cypress, cassia, geranium, lavender, manuka, marjoram, melaleuca, myrrh, oregano, peppermint, rosemary, tea tree, thyme

# Problem Search S

**SCALP CONDITIONS:** *Bay West Indies, manuka, rosemary, ylang-ylang*

**SCARS:** *benzoin, carrot seed, cistus, elemi, frankincense, geranium, helichrysum, jasmine, lavender, mandarin, myrrh, palmarosa, patchouli, rose, sandalwood*

**SCIATICA:** *(also see neuropathy) balsam fir, blue tansy, cardamom, helichrysum, lavender, peppermint, Roman chamomile, sandalwood, St. John's wort, tansy, tarragon, thyme, white fir, wintergreen*

**SCRAPES:** *(see cuts) basil, clary sage, cypress, frankincense, helichrysum, lavender, lemon, lemongrass, melaleuca, peppermint, Roman chamomile*

**SCURVY:** *citrus oils, ginger*

**SEDATIVE:** *clary sage, cypress, fennel, frankincense, lavender, marjoram, melissa, myrrh, orange, patchouli, peppermint, Roman chamomile, rosemary, sandalwood, vetiver, white fir, ylang-ylang*

**SEIZURES:** *clary sage, lavender, melissa, orange, sandalwood, vetiver*

**SEXUAL ENHANCEMENT:** *amyris, cilantro, cinnamon, clary sage, cypress, fennel, frankincense, geranium, ginger, grapefruit, jasmine, lavender, myrrh, neroli, nutmeg, orange, patchouli, pimento, rose, rosewood, sandalwood, thyme, vanilla, ylang-ylang*

**SHINGLES:** *(see viruses) bergamot, eucalyptus, geranium, lavender, lemon, melaleuca, Roman chamomile*

**SHOCK:** *basil, cilantro, helichrysum, melaleuca, melissa, myrrh, orange, peppermint, Roman chamomile, rosemary, ylang-ylang*

**SINUS CONGESTION/PLUGGED:** *balsam fir, basil, cajeput, cardamom, cedarwood, clove, elemi, eucalyptus, ginger, helichrysum, melaleuca, niaouli, peppermint, pine, ravensara, white fir*

**SKIN HEALTH:** Bay West Indies, benzoin, bergamot, blue cypress, blue tansy, cajeput, carrot seed, cassia, cedarwood, cypress, frankincense, galbanum, geranium, German chamomile, helichrysum, juniper, lavender, lemon, lovage leaf, mandarin, manuka, marjoram, melaleuca, myrrh, myrtle, orange, patchouli, peppermint, Roman chamomile, rosemary, sandalwood, vetiver, ylang-ylang

**SMELL IMPROVEMENT:** basil, peppermint

**SNAKE BITE:** basil, cinnamon, clove, frankincense, helichrysum, lavender, lemon, melaleuca, tea tree, thyme

**SORE THROAT:** basil, bergamot, cassia, cinnamon, clary sage, clove, cypress, eucalyptus, frankincense, geranium, ginger, grapefruit, helichrysum, lavender, lemon, lemongrass, marjoram, melaleuca, myrrh, orange, oregano, peppermint, Roman chamomile, rosemary, sandalwood, thyme, white fir, wintergreen

**SPASMS:** (see muscle aches/spasms) basil, catnip, cypress, lavender, marjoram, oregano, peppermint, Roman chamomile, thyme, valerian

**SPIDER BITES:** basil, cinnamon, cypress, helichrysum, lavender, lemon, lemongrass, oregano, peppermint, tea tree, thyme

**SPIDER VEINS:** basil, chamomile, citrus oils, cypress, eucalyptus, fennel, geranium, grape seed oil, grapefruit, helichrysum, juniper, lavender, lemon, lemongrass, lime, marjoram, orange, peppermint, rosemary

**SPLEEN:** basil, bergamot, cinnamon, clary sage, clove, cypress, eucalyptus, frankincense, ginger, lavender, lemon, marjoram, melaleuca, myrrh, orange, oregano, peppermint, Roman chamomile, rosemary, sandalwood, thyme, thyme, white fir, wintergreen

**SPLINTER/SLIVER:** helichrysum, lavender

**SPRAINS/STRAINS:** basil, blue tansy, cypress, ginger, helichrysum, jasmine, lavender, lemongrass, marjoram, peppermint, rosemary, thyme, vetiver, white fir, wintergreen

**STAPH INFECTION:** (see bacterial infections) geranium, helichrysum, melaleuca, oregano, thyme

**STIMULANT:** (see alertness) *basil, eucalyptus, ginger, grapefruit, orange, peppermint, rose, rosemary*

**STREP INFECTION:** *basil, bergamot, cinnamon, clary sage, clove, cypress, eucalyptus, frankincense, ginger, lavender, lemon, marjoram, melaleuca, myrrh, orange, oregano, peppermint, Roman chamomile, rosemary, sandalwood, thyme, white fir, wintergreen*

**STREP THROAT/TONSILLITIS:** *basil, cassia, cinnamon, clary sage, clove, cypress, eucalyptus, frankincense, geranium, grapefruit, helichrysum, lavender, lemon, lemongrass, marjoram, melaleuca, oregano, peppermint, rosemary, thyme*

**STRESS:** *angelica, anise seed, balsam fir, basil, benzoin, bergamot, blue tansy, cilantro, cinnamon, clary sage, clove, coriander, cypress, davana, elemi, fennel, frankincense, geranium, grapefruit, ho wood, hops, juniper, lavender, lemon, lemongrass, lime, mandarin, marjoram, melissa, orange, patchouli, peppermint, petitgrain, pimento, Roman chamomile, rose, rosemary, sandalwood, spikenard, St. John's wort, thyme, valerian, vetiver, white fir, ylang-ylang*

**STRETCH MARKS:** *frankincense, galbanum, geranium, helichrysum, jasmine, lavandin, lavender, myrrh, neroli, rose, ylang-ylang*

**STROKE/CVA:** *cilantro, cypress, fennel, helichrysum*

**STUBBED TOE:** (see pain or inflammation) *marjoram, peppermint*

**SUNBURN:** *basil, blue tansy, carrot seed, cypress, geranium, helichrysum, lavender, melaleuca, peppermint, Roman chamomile, St. John's wort*

**SWEATING:** *chamomile, cypress, geranium, lavender, lemon, peppermint, sage, tea tree*

# Problem Search T-Z

**TEETH CARE/PAIN/HEALING:** *basil, clove, fennel, ginger, helichrysum, lavender, melaleuca, myrrh, orange, peppermint, Roman chamomile*

**TEETHING PAIN:** *German chamomile, Roman chamomile*

**TENNIS ELBOW:** (see inflammation) *eucalyptus, helichrysum, lemongrass, peppermint, wintergreen*

**TENSION:** *balsam fir, basil, benzoin, bergamot, clary sage, coriander, eucalyptus, frankincense, grapefruit, helichrysum, jasmine, lemongrass, marjoram, peppermint, Roman chamomile, wintergreen, ylang-ylang*

**THRUSH/ORAL CANDIDA:** (see fungal infections) *geranium, lavender, lemon, melaleuca, thyme*

**TICKS:** (see parasites) *lavender, peppermint, oregano, thyme*

**TONSILLITIS:** *basil, cassia, cinnamon, clary sage, clove, cypress, eucalyptus, frankincense, geranium, grapefruit, helichrysum, lavender, lemon, lemongrass, marjoram, melaleuca, oregano, peppermint, rosemary, thyme*

**TOOTHACHE:** *basil, cajeput, clove, German chamomile, helichrysum, lavandin, lavender, melaleuca, orange, peppermint, Roman chamomile, tansy*

**TUMORS:** *clove, frankincense, grapefruit, helichrysum, lavender, sandalwood*

**ULCERS-GASTRIC:** (see indigestion) *bergamot, cinnamon, fennel, frankincense, geranium, ginger, orange, peppermint, rose, sage*

**URINARY TRACT HEALTH:** *cypress, eucalyptus, geranium, lavender, lemon, lime, melaleuca, orange, peppermint, rosemary, sandalwood, thyme*

**URINARY TRACT INFECTION:** balsam fir, bergamot, cedarwood, celery seed, copaiba, cypress, eucalyptus, geranium, lavender, lemon, lime, melaleuca, mountain savory, orange, peppermint, rosemary, sandalwood, tarragon, thyme

**VAGINAL INFECTION:** eucalyptus, mountain savory

**VAGINAL CANDIDA:** basil, clary, cypress, eucalyptus, geranium, lavender, lemon, melaleuca, rosemary, thyme

**VARICOSE VEINS:** basil, bergamot, cypress, geranium, helichrysum, lavender, lemon, lemongrass, orange, peppermint, rosemary, St. John's wort, vanilla, yarrow

**VERTIGO:** basil, geranium, ginger, helichrysum, lavender

**VIRUSES:** basil, bay laurel, bergamot, black spruce, blue cypress, cassia, cinnamon, clary sage, clove, cypress, eucalyptus, frankincense, geranium, ginger, grapefruit, helichrysum, hyssop, Idaho blue spruce, lavender, lemon, lemongrass, marjoram, melaleuca, melissa, myrrh, orange, oregano, peppermint, Roman chamomile, rosemary, sandalwood, thyme, white fir, wintergreen

**VOMITING:** cajeput, cardamom, cinnamon, fennel, ginger, lavender, oregano, peppermint, pimento, Roman chamomile, rose, thyme

**WARTS:** cinnamon, clove, cypress, frankincense, helichrysum, lavender, lemon, melaleuca, oregano, tea tree, thyme

**WATER RETENTION:** angelica, carrot seed, cypress, geranium, grapefruit, grapefruit, hyssop, juniper, lemon, lemongrass, rosemary, tangerine

**WEIGHT INCREASE/GAIN DESIRED:** (see anorexia and bulimia)

**WEIGHT LOSS:** bitter orange, cistus oils, fennel, frankincense, ginger, grapefruit, lavender, ledum, lemon, orange, peppermint, rosemary, thyme

**WHIPLASH:** (see inflammation or muscle aches) basil, birch, clove, helichrysum, lemongrass, marjoram, Roman chamomile, vetiver

**WOUNDS:** *balsam fir, basil, benzoin, bergamot, black spruce, carrot seed, cistus, clary sage, clove, cypress, dill, eucalyptus, fir needle, frankincense, geranium, helichrysum, lavender, lemon, lemongrass, melaleuca, myrrh, niaouli, oak moss, patchouli, peppermint, Roman chamomile, rose, sandalwood, tagetes, tea tree, thyme, yarrow*

**WRINKLES:** *carrot seed, cistus, clary sage, cypress, elemi, fennel, frankincense, galbanum, geranium, helichrysum, lavender, lemon lime, lemon, mandarin, myrrh, myrtle, neroli, orange, oregano, palmarosa, patchouli, rose, rosemary, sandalwood, thyme, ylang-ylang*

**YEAST INFECTION/CANDIDA:** *blue cypress, clove, elemi, eucalyptus, lavender, lemon, melaleuca, myrrh, oregano, palmarosa, patchouli, peppermint, rosemary, thyme*

# Oil Search A-B

**ALLSPICE:** analgesic, anesthetic, antibacterial, antifungal, antioxidant, antiseptic, antiviral, aphrodisiac, carminative, rubefacient, stimulant.
***Blends well with*-**bay, bergamot, black pepper, cistus, coriander, geranium, ginger, lavender, neroli, orange, patchouli, ylang-ylang

**AMYRIS:** antiseptic, balsamic, decongestant, emollient, muscle-relaxant, sedative.
***Blends well with*-**cedarwood, citronella, ginger, ho wood, lavender, oak moss, balsam and ylang-ylang

**ANGELICA:** antibacterial, antifungal, antiseptic, antispasmodic, carminative, cholagogue, depurative, diaphoretic, digestive, diuretic, emmenagogue, expectorant, febrifuge, nervine, stimulant, stomachic, tonic.
***Blends well with*-**citrus oils, cedarwood, clary sage, oakmoss, patchouli, vetiver.

**ANISE SEED:** analgesic, antiseptic, antispasmodic, aperitive, carminative, digestive, diuretic, emmenagogue, expectorant, stimulant, stomachic.
***Blends well with*-**bay, black pepper, ginger, lavender, orange, pine, rose.

**BALSAM FIR:** anticoagulant, antiinflammatory, antiseptic, astringent, expectorant, sedative, tonic.
***Blends well with*-**Douglas fir, white fir, spruce and pine.

**BASIL:** analgesic, antibacterial, antidepressant, antiinflammatory, antiseptic, antispasmodic, carminative, cephalic, digestive, emmenagogue, expectorant, febrifuge, nervine, stimulant, stomachic, sudorific, tonic.
***Blends well with*-**bergamot, citronella, citrus oils, clary sage, geranium, hyssop, rosemary.

**BAY LAUREL:** analgesic, anesthetic, antibacterial, anticonvulsant, antifungal, antimicrobial, antirheumatic, antiseptic, aperitive, carminative, diaphoretic, diuretic, expectorant, sedative.

***Blends well with*-**bergamot, clary sage, cypress, frankincense, ginger, juniper, lavender, orange, patchouli, pine, rosemary, ylang-ylang.

**BAY WEST INDIES:** analgesic, anticonvulsant, antineuralgic, antiseptic, astringent, expectorant, hair, tonic, stimulant.
***Blends well with*-**bergamot, black pepper, cardamom, cinnamon, clove, coriander, frankincense, geranium, ginger, lavender, grapefruit, lemon, mandarin, petitgrain, rosemary, sandalwood, ylang-ylang.

**BENZOIN:** antidepressant, antiinflammatory, antimicrobial, antiseptic, astringent, carminative, diuretic, expectorant, sedative, vulnerary, warming.
***Blends well with*-**bergamot, black pepper, copaiba balsam, coriander, cypress, frankincense, ginger, jasmine, juniper, lemon, myrrh, petitgrain, rose, sandalwood.

**BERGAMOT:** analgesic, anthelmintic, antibacterial, antidepressant, antiseptic, antispasmodic, antiviral, astringent, carminative, cicatrizant, cooling, digestive, diuretic, expectorant, febrifuge, laxative, rubefacient, sedative, stimulant, stomachic, tonic, vermifuge, vulnerary.
***Blends well with*-**chamomile, citrus oils, coriander, cypress, geranium, helichrysum, jasmine, juniper, lavender, lemon balm, neroli, nutmeg, rose, sandalwood, vetiver, violet, ylang-ylang

**BIRCH:** analgesic, antiinflammatory, antiseptic, depurative, disinfectant, diuretic, febrifuge, insecticide, tonic, warming.
***Blends well with*-**benzoin, sandalwood, rosemary, jasmine.

**BLACK PEPPER:** analgesic, antibacterial, antifungal, antimicrobial, antiseptic, antispasmodic, aperitive, carminative, diaphoretic, digestive, diuretic, febrifuge, laxative, rubefacient, stimulant, stomachic, tonic, vasodilator.
***Blends well with*-**cardamom, clary sage, clove, frankincense, geranium, lavender, juniper, marjoram, myrrh, orange, nutmeg, rosemary, sage, sandalwood, tea tree, vetiver, ylang-ylang.

**BLUE CYPRESS:** antiinflammatory, antiviral, insect-repellent, stimulant.
***Blends well with*-**cardamom, cedarwood, clary sage, geranium, jasmine, myrtle, sandalwood, pine, rose, lavender, orange, tea tree.

**BLUE TANSY:** analgesic, anesthetic, antibacterial, antihistamine, antiinflammatory, anti-itch, hypotensive, nervine, relaxant.
***Blends well with*-**cedarwood, cistus, helichrysum, lavender, rosemary, ravensara.

# Oil Search C

**CAJEPUT:** analgesic, antibacterial, antimicrobial, antineuralgic, antiseptic, antispasmodic, carminative, decongestant, diaphoretic, expectorant, febrifuge, insecticide, stimulant, sudorific, tonic, vermifuge, vulnerary.
***Blends well with-***angelica, cedarwood, clary sage, clove, geranium, lavender, marjoram, oak moss, pine, rosemary, allspice, thyme, ylang-ylang.

**CAMPHOR:** analgesic, antiinflammatory, antiseptic, antispasmodic, antiviral, bactericidal, decongestant, diuretic, expectorant, rubefacient, stimulant, sudorific, vermifuge, vulnerary.
***Blends well with-***basil, cajeput, chamomile, citrus oils, eucalyptus, lavender, rosemary, allspice.

**CARDAMOM:** antibacterial, antiseptic, antispasmodic, aphrodisiac, carminative, cephalic, digestive, diuretic, laxative, nerve, stimulant, stomachic, tonic.
***Blends well with-***bay, bergamot, black pepper, cedarwood, cinnamon, clove, coriander, fennel, ginger, grapefruit, jasmine, lemon, lemongrass, neroli, orange, patchouli, petitgrain, sandalwood, ylang-ylang.

**CARROT SEED:** anthelmintic, antiseptic, carminative, cytophylactic, depurative, diuretic, emmenagogue, hepatic, stimulant, tonic, vermifuge.
***Blends well with-***allspice, cassia, cedarwood, cinnamon, citrus oils, fennel, frankincense, geranium.

**CASSIA:** antiarthritic, antidepressant, antidiarrheal, antiemetic, anti-galactagogue, antimicrobial, antirheumatic, antiviral, astringent, carminative, circulatory, emmenagogue, febrifuge, stimulant.
***Blends well with-***balsam oils, black pepper, chamomile, coriander, frankincense, ginger, geranium, nutmeg, rosemary, citrus oils.

**CATNIP:** anesthetic, antiinflammatory, antirheumatic, antispasmodic, astringent, carminative, diaphoretic, insecticide, nervine, sedative, tonic.

***Blends well with*-**grapefruit, lavender, lemon, marjoram, peppermint, orange, rosemary, spearmint

**CEDARWOOD:** antifungal, antiseborrheic, antiseptic, antispasmodic, astringent, circulatory, diaphoretic, diuretic, emmenagogue, expectorant, fungicidal, insecticide, sedative, tonic.
***Blends well with*-**bergamot, cassia, chamomile, clary sage, cypress, eucalyptus, jasmine, juniper, lavender, neroli, palmarosa, petitgrain, rosemary, sandalwood, vetiver, ylang-ylang.

**CELERY SEED:** antirheumatic, antiseptic, antispasmodic, carminative, digestive, diuretic, emmenagogue, galactagogue, hepatic, nervine, sedative, stomachic, tonic.
***Blends well with*-**black pepper, coriander, ginger, lavender, lovage, oakmoss, pine, tea tree.

**CHAMOMILE-GERMAN:** analgesic, antiinflammatory, antiphlogistic, antispasmodic, bactericidal, carminative, cicatrizant, digestive, emmenagogue, febrifuge, fungicidal, hepatic, nervine, stomachic, sudorific, vermifuge, vulnerary.
***Blends well with*-**bergamot, citrus oils, clary sage, frankincense, geranium, grapefruit, jasmine, lavender, lemon, lime, marjoram, neroli, patchouli, rose, rosemary, tea tree, ylang-ylang.

**CHAMOMILE-ROMAN:** analgesic, antibacterial, antiinflammatory, antiinflammatory, antimicrobial, antineuralgic, antiphlogistic, antiseptic, antispasmodic, bactericidal, carminative, cholagogue, digestive, emmenagogue, febrifuge, hepatic, nervine, sedative, stomachic, sudorific, tonic, vermifuge, vulnerary.
***Blends well with*-**bergamot, clary sage, eucalyptus, geranium, grapefruit, jasmine, lavender, lemon, neroli, oakmoss, rose, tea tree.

**CILANTRO:** analgesic, antiinflammatory, antioxidant, antispasmodic, aperitive, bactericidal, cardamom, depurative, digestive, fungicidal, stimulant, stomachic.
***Blends well with*-**bergamot, cinnamon, citronella, clary sage, cypress, frankincense, ginger, jasmine, neroli, petitgrain, pine, sandalwood, spice oils.

**CINNAMON:** analgesic, antibacterial, anticoagulant, antifungal, antiinflammatory, antimicrobial, antiseptic, antispasmodic, astringent, carminative, digestive, expectorant, stimulant, stomachic, tree, vermifuge.

***Blends well with*-**bergamot, cardamom, clove, frankincense, ginger, grapefruit, lemon, marjoram, orange, peppermint, rose, vanilla, ylang-ylang.

**CISTUS:** antimicrobial, antiseptic, astringent, emmenagogue, expectorant, tonic.
***Blends well with*-**bergamot, chamomile, clary sage, cypress, frankincense, lavender, juniper, oakmoss, patchouli, pine, sandalwood, vetiver.

**CITRONELLA:** analgesic, antibacterial, antifungal, antiseptic, antispasmodic, astringent, diaphoretic, diuretic, emmenagogue, febrifuge, fungicidal, sedative's, stimulant, stomachic, tonic.
***Blends well with*-**bergamot, cedarwood, citrus oils, geranium, pine, sandalwood.

**CLARY SAGE:** antibacterial, antidepressant, antiinflammatory, antiphlogistic, antiseptic, antispasmodic, aphrodisiac, astringent, carminative, digestive, emmenagogue, hypotensive, nervine, relaxant, sedative, stomachic, tonic, vulnerary, warming.
***Blends well with*-**bergamot, black pepper, cardamom, cedarwood, chamomile, cypress, frankincense, geranium, grapefruit, jasmine, juniper, lavender, lemon balm, line, patchouli, rose, sandalwood, tea tree.

**CLOVE:** analgesic, antiaging, antibacterial, anticoagulant, antifungal, antiinflammatory, antimicrobial, antioxidant, antiseptic, antispasmodic, antiviral, carminative, expectorant, insecticide, stimulant.
***Blends well with*-**allspice, bay, bergamot, chamomile, clary sage, geranium, ginger, grapefruit, jasmine, lavender, lemon, mandarin, palmarosa, rose, sandalwood, vanilla, ylang-ylang**.

**COPAIBA:** analgesic, antibacterial, antiinflammatory, antiseptic, disinfectant, diuretic, expectorant, stimulant.
***Blends well with*-**allspice, cedarwood, citrus oils, clary sage, frankincense, jasmine, rose, sandalwood, vanilla, ylang-ylang

**CORIANDER:** analgesic, antispasmodic, aphrodisiac, bactericidal, carminative, depurative, digestive, fungicidal, lipolytic, stimulant, stomachic.
***Blends well with*-**bergamot, black pepper, cardamom, cinnamon, clary sage, clove, cypress, frankincense, geranium, ginger, grapefruit,

jasmine, lemon, neroli, orange, palmarosa, pine, sandalwood, ylang-ylang.

**CORNMINT:** anesthetic, antimicrobial, antiseptic, antispasmodic, carminative, digestive, expectorant, stimulant, stomachic.
**Blends well with**-basil, benzoin, black pepper, cypress, eucalyptus, geranium, grapefruit, juniper, lavender, lemon, marjoram, niaouli, pine, ravensara, rosemary, tea tree.

**CYPRESS:** antibacterial, antiinflammatory, antiseptic, antispasmodic, astringent, diuretic, emmenagogue, expectorant, febrifuge, hemostatic, hepatic, insecticide, sedative, sudorific, tonic, vasoconstrictor.
**Blends well with**-black pepper, cedarwood, chamomile, citrus oils, clary sage, ginger, lavender, pine, ylang-ylang.

# Oil Search D-G

**DAVANA:** antiseptic, antiviral, aphrodisiac, disinfectant, emmenagogue, expectorant, nervine, sedative, vulnerary.
***Blends well with*-**amyris, bergamot, black pepper, cardamom, chamomile, jasmine, mandarin, neroli, orange, patchouli, rose, sandalwood, spikenard, tangerine, vanilla, ylang-ylang.

**DILL SEED:** antispasmodic, bactericidal, carminative, digestive, emmenagogue, hypotensive, stimulant, stomachic.
***Blends well with*-**black pepper, cinnamon, citrus oils, clove, nutmeg, peppermint, spearmint.

**DORADO AZIL:** analgesic, anticancer, antifungal, antiinfectious, antiinflammatory, antimicrobial, antioxidant, insecticide.
***Blends well with*-**balsam fir, copaiba, elemi, eucalyptus, helichrysum, lavender, wintergreen.

**DOUGLAS FIR:** antiseptic, antifungal, antitussive, calmative, disinfectant, expectorant, nervine, stomachic, tonic, vasodilator.
***Blends well with*-**cistus, other fir oils, lavender, lemon, marjoram, pine, rosemary.

**ELEMI:** analgesic, antiseptic, antiviral, cicatrizant, expectorant, fungicidal, stimulant, stomachic, tonic.
***Blends well with*-**cinnamon, frankincense, lavender, myrrh, rosemary, sage, spice oils.

**EUCALYPTUS:** analgesic, antibacterial, antifungal, antiinflammatory, antineuralgic, antirheumatic, antiseptic, antispasmodic, antiviral, astringent, cicatrizant, decongestant, depurative, diuretic, expectorant, febrifuge, insecticide, rubefacient, stimulant, vermifuge, vulnerary.
***Blends well with*-**cedarwood, chamomile, geranium, ginger, grapefruit, lavender, lemon, marjoram, peppermint, pine, rosemary, thyme.

**FENNEL:** analgesic, anesthetic, antimicrobial, antiseptic, antispasmodic, aperitive, carminative, depurative, diuretic,

emmenagogue, expectorant, galactagogue, laxative, splenic, stimulant, stomachic, tonic, vermifuge.
**Blends well with-**bergamot, black pepper, cardamom, cypress, dill, for, geranium, ginger, grapefruit, juniper, lavender, lemon, mandarin, marjoram, niaouli, orange, pine, ravensara, rose, rosemary, sandalwood, tangerine, ylang-ylang.

**FIR NEEDLE:** analgesic, antiseptic, antitussive, astringent, expectorant, rubefacient, stimulant, tonic.
**Blends well with-**benzoin, cistus, lavender, lemon, marjoram, orange, pine, rosemary.

**FRANKINCENSE:** analgesic, anticatarrhal, antidepressant, antifungal, antiinflammatory, antioxidant, antiseptic, antitussive, astringent, calming, carminative, cicatrizant, cytophylactic, digestive, diuretic, emmenagogue, expectorant, rubefacient, sedative, tonic, uterine, vulnerary.
**Blends well with-**bergamot, black pepper, cinnamon, cypress, geranium, grapefruit, lavender, lemon, mandarin, neroli, orange, patchouli, pine, rose, sandalwood, vetiver, ylang-ylang.

**GALBANUM:** analgesic, antiinflammatory, antimicrobial, antiseptic, antispasmodic, balsamic, carminative, digestive, diuretic, emmenagogue, expectorant, hypotensive, tonic.
**Blends well with-**benzoin, fir oils, geranium, ginger, lavender, oakmoss, pine.

**GERANIUM:** analgesic, antibacterial, antidepressant, antidiabetic, antiinflammatory, antiinflammatory, antiseptic, astringent, cicatrizant, cytophylactic, diuretic, emmenagogue, hemostatic, hepatic, insecticide, rubefacient, sedative, stimulant, styptic, tonic, vasoconstrictor, vermifuge, vulnerary.
**Blends well with-**bergamot, chamomile, clary sage, clove, cypress, ginger, grapefruit, jasmine, juniper, lemon, mandarin, neroli, palmarosa, patchouli, peppermint, rose, rosemary, sandalwood, ylang-ylang.

**GINGER:** analgesic, antibacterial, anticoagulant, antiinflammatory, antioxidant, antiseptic, antispasmodic, aperitive, aphrodisiac's, carminative, cephalic, cholagogue, diaphoretic, digestive, diuretic, expectorant, febrifuge, laxative, rubefacient, stimulant, stomachic, sudorific, tonic, warming.

***Blends well with***-bergamot, cedarwood, clove, eucalyptus, frankincense, geranium, grapefruit, jasmine, lemon, neroli, orange, patchouli, rose, sandalwood, ylang-ylang.

**GOLDENROD:** antiinflammatory, anti-hypertensive, diuretic, liver, stimulant.
***Blends well with***-balsam oils, ginger, spruce.

**GRAPEFRUIT:** antibacterial, antidepressant, antiseptic, astringent, depurative, digestive, disinfectant, diuretic, stimulant, tonic.
***Blends well with***-bergamot, black pepper, cardamom, clary sage, clove, cypress, eucalyptus, frankincense, geranium, ginger, juniper, lavender, lemon, mandarin, neroli, patchouli, peppermint, rosemary, ylang-ylang.

# Oil Search H-L

**HELICHRYSUM:** antibacterial, antiinflammatory, antiinflammatory, antimicrobial, antioxidant, antiseptic, antispasmodic, astringent, cholagogue, cicatrizant, diuretic, expectorant, hepatic, mucolytic, nervine, stimulant.
***Blends well with*-**bergamot, black pepper, chamomile, citrus oils, clary sage, clove, cypress, geranium, juniper, lavender, neroli, rose, rosemary, tea tree, thyme, ylang-ylang.

**HINOKI:** antibacterial, antifungal, antiinfectious, antimicrobial, antiseptic, antiviral, astringent, decongestant, insecticide, mucolytic, relaxant.
***Blends well with*-**cypress, jasmine, ylang-ylang.

**HO WOOD:** analgesic, antiseptic, sedative.
***Blends well with*-**basil, cajeput, chamomile, lavender, sandalwood, ylang-ylang.

**HOPS:** antimicrobial, antiseptic, antispasmodic, astringent, bactericidal, carminative, diuretic, nervine, sedative.
***Blends well with*-**balsam, citrus oils, copaiba, nutmeg, pine, spice oils.

**HYSSOP:** antibacterial, antirheumatic, antiseptic, antispasmodic, antiviral, astringent, carminative, cephalic, cicatrizant, digestive, diuretic, emmenagogue, expectorant, febrifuge, hypertensive, nervine, sedative, stimulant, sudorific, tonic, vermifuge, vulnerary.
***Blends well with*-**angelica, clary sage, geranium, hyssop, lavandin, lavender, lemon, myrtle, orange, rosemary, sage.

**IDAHO BLUE, SPRUCE:** antibacterial, anticancer, antiinfectious, antiinflammatory, antiseptic, antispasmodic, antiviral, disinfectant, expectorant, immunostimulant.
***Blends well with*-**balsam fir, bergamot, coriander, frankincense, geranium, myrrh, thyme, ylang-ylang.

**JASMINE:** analgesic, antidepressant, antiinflammatory, antiseptic, antispasmodic, aphrodisiac, carminative, emmenagogue, expectorant, galactagogue, relaxant, sedative, tonic, uterine.

***Blends well with*-**bergamot, clary sage, clove, coriander, ginger, grapefruit, lemon, mandarin, neroli, orange, palmarosa, patchouli, petitgrain, rose, sandalwood, ylang-ylang.

**JUNIPER BERRY:** analgesic, antimicrobial, antiputrefactive, antirheumatic, antiseptic, antispasmodic, astringent, carminative, depurative, detoxicant, digestive, diuretic, emmenagogue, relaxant, rubefacient, sedative, stimulant, stomachic, sudorific, tonic, vulnerary.
***Blends well with*-**bergamot, black pepper,cedarwood, clary sage, cypress, elemi, fir needle, grapefruit, lavender, lavandin, lemon, lime, lemongrass, oakmoss, rosemary, vetiver.

**LAVANDIN:** antidepressant, antiseptic, analgesic, cicatrizant, expectorant, nervine, vulnerary.
***Blends well with*-**bergamot, citronella, lemongrass, cinnamon, rosemary, pine, jasmine, thyme, patchouli.

**LAVENDER:** analgesic, antibacterial, antidepressant, antiinflammatory, antimicrobial, antirheumatic, antiseptic, antispasmodic, antiviral, bactericidal, calming, carminative, cholagogue, cicatrizant, cytophylactic, decongestant, diuretic, emmenagogue, fungicidal, hypotensive, insecticide, nervine, relaxant, sedative, stimulant, stomachic, sudorific, vulnerary.
***Blends well with*-**bergamot, black pepper, cedarwood, chamomile, clary sage, clove, cypress, eucalyptus, geranium, grapefruit, juniper, lemon, lemongrass, mandarin, marjoram, patchouli, peppermint, pine, rose, rosemary, tea tree, thyme, vetiver.

**LEDUM:** antibacterial, anticancer, antiviral, antiinflammatory, nerve-stimulant, tonic, diuretic.
***Blends well with*-**celery seed, fennel, grapefruit, helichrysum, hyssop, lemon, petitgrain, ravensara, spearmint, wintergreen.

**LEMON:** antibacterial, antifungal, antiinflammatory, antimicrobial, antirheumatic, antiseptic, antispasmodic, astringent, carminative, cicatrizant, depurative, diaphoretic, digestive, diuretic, hypotensive, insecticide, laxative, rubefacient, sedative, tonic, vermifuge.
***Blends well with*-**chamomile, elemi, eucalyptus, fennel, frankincense, geranium, juniper, lavender, niaouli, oakmoss, rose, sandalwood, ylang-ylang, other citrus oils.

**LEMON BALM (MELISSA):** antibacterial, antihistamine, antiinflammatory, antiseptic, antispasmodic, antiviral, bactericidal, carminative, diaphoretic, digestive, emmenagogue, febrifuge, nervine, sedative, tonic, vermifuge.
***Blends well with*-**citrus oils, chamomile, frankincense, geranium, lavender, neroli, petitgrain, rose.

**LEMONGRASS:** analgesic, antidepressant, antifungal, antiinflammatory, antimicrobial, antioxidant, antiparasitic, antiseptic, antiviral, astringent, bactericidal, carminative, digestive, febrifuge, fungicidal, fungicidal:, insecticide, nervine, sedative, stimulant, tonic.
***Blends well with*-**basil, bergamot, black pepper, cedarwood, clary sage, cypress, fennel, geranium, ginger, grapefruit, lavender, lemon, marjoram, orange, patchouli, rosemary, tea tree, thyme, ylang-ylang.

**LIME:** antibacterial, antiseptic, antispasmodic, antiviral, aperitive, astringent, bactericidal, carminative, disinfectant, febrifuge, hemostatic, insecticide, tonic.
***Blends well with*-**citronella, clary sage, lavender, neroli, nutmeg, rosemary, vanilla, ylang-ylang.

**LITSEA CUBEBA:** antibiotic, antiinfectious, antiinflammatory, antiseptic, digestive, insecticide, sedative, stimulant, stomachic, vulnerary.
***Blends well with*-**basil, bay, black pepper, cardamom, cedarwood, chamomile, clary sage, coriander, cypress, eucalyptus, frankincense, geranium, ginger, grapefruit, juniper, marjoram, orange, palmarosa, patchouli, petitgrain, rosemary, sandalwood, tea tree, thyme, vetiver, ylang-ylang.

**LOVAGE LEAF:** antimicrobial, antiseptic, antispasmodic, carminative, diaphoretic, digestive, diuretic, emmenagogue, expectorant, febrifuge, stimulant, stomachic.
***Blends well with*-**bay, galbanum, lavender, marjoram, oakmoss, rose, spice oils.

# Oil Search M-P

**MACE:** analgesic, antioxidant, antispasmodic, aphrodisiac, carminative, cholagogue, laxative, stimulant, tonic.
***Blends well with*-**bay, citrus oils, clary sage, geranium, lavender, lime, oakmoss, rosemary, neroli.

**MANDARIN:** antiseptic, antispasmodic, antiviral, carminative, cholagogue, depurative, digestive, diuretic, hypnotic, laxative, lymphatic-stimulant, sedative, tonic.
***Blends well with*-**basil, black pepper, cinnamon, clary sage, clove, frankincense, geranium, grapefruit, jasmine, juniper, lemon, marjoram, neroli, nutmeg, palmarosa, patchouli, petitgrain, roman chamomile, rose, sandalwood, ylang-ylang.

**MANUKA:** analgesic, anesthetic, antibacterial, antifungal, antiinflammatory, antimicrobial, antiseptic, antiviral, expectorant, immunostimulant, insecticide, nervine, sedative, vulnerary.
***Blends well with*-**basil, bergamot, black pepper, chamomile, clary sage, cypress, eucalyptus, geranium, grapefruit, lavender, lemon, litsea cubeba, marjoram, orange, patchouli, peppermint, petitgrain, pine, ravensara, rosemary, sage, sandalwood, tea tree, thyme.

**MARJORAM:** analgesic, anaphrodisiac, antioxidant, antiseptic, antispasmodic, antiviral, bactericidal, carminative, cephalic, diaphoretic, digestive, diuretic, emmenagogue, expectorant, fungicidal, hypotensive, laxative, nervine, relaxant, sedative, stomachic, tonic, vasodilator, vulnerary, warming.
***Blends well with*-**basil, bergamot, black pepper, cedarwood, chamomile, cypress, eucalyptus, lemon, fennel, juniper, lavender, lemon, orange, peppermint, pine, rosemary, tea tree, thyme.

**MELALEUCA/TEA TREE:** (see, tea, tree)

**MELISSA: (see lemon balm)** antidepressant, antispasmodic, antiviral, bactericidal, carminative, diaphoretic, emmenagogue, febrifuge, hypotensive, nervine, sedative, stomachic, sudorific, tonic.

**MOUNTAIN SAVORY:** antibacterial, antifungal, antiinflammatory, antiinfectious, antiparasitic, antiviral, immunostimulant.

***Blends well with*-**lemon, oregano.

**MYRRH:** anticatarrhal, antifungal, antiinflammatory, antimicrobial, antiseptic, antispasmodic, antiviral, astringent, carminative, cicatrizant, digestive, emmenagogue, expectorant, fungicidal, sedative, stomachic, tonic, uterine, vulnerary.
***Blends well with*-**bergamot, chamomile, clove, cypress, eucalyptus, lemon, frankincense, geranium, grapefruit, jasmine, juniper, lavender, lemon, neroli, patchouli, pine, rose, rosemary, sandalwood, tea tree, ylang-ylang.

**MYRTLE:** antibacterial, anticatarrhal, antiseptic, astringent, bactericidal, expectorant, sedative, tonic.
***Blends well with*-**bergamot, black pepper, clary sage, clove, ginger, hyssop, lavender, lime, rosemary.

**NEROLI:** antibacterial, antidepressant, antiinflammatory, antiinflammatory, antiseptic, antispasmodic, aphrodisiac, carminative, cicatrizant, digestive, fungicidal, nervine, sedative, tonic.
***Blends well with*-**benzoin, chamomile, clary sage, contents, geranium, ginger, grapefruit, jasmine, juniper, lavender, lemon, orange, rose, rosemary, sandalwood, ylang-ylang.

**NIAOULI:** analgesic, anticatarrhal, antirheumatic, antiseptic, antispasmodic, bactericidal, cicatrizant, decongestant, diaphoretic, expectorant, febrifuge, insecticide, stimulant, vermifuge, vulnerary.
***Blends well with*-**bergamot, eucalyptus, lavender, lemon, orange, tea tree.

**NUTMEG:** analgesic, antiinflammatory, antioxidant, antirheumatic, antiseptic, antispasmodic, aperitive, aphrodisiac, carminative, cholagogue, digestive, emmenagogue, laxative, stimulant, tonic.
***Blends well with*-**bay, clary sage, coriander, geranium, lavender, lime, mandarin, oakmoss, orange, balsam, petitgrain, rosemary.

**OAK MOSS:** antiseptic, demulcent, expectorant, fixative.
***Blends well with*-**anise, bay, bergamot, clary sage, cypress, eucalyptus, ginger, lavender, lime, orange, palmarosa, tea tree, vetiver, ylang-ylang.

**ORANGE/BITTER:** antidepressant, antiinflammatory, antiseptic, antispasmodic, astringent, bactericidal, carminative, digestive, fungicidal, sedative, stimulant, stomachic, tonic.

**Blends well with**-clary sage, clove, cinnamon, frankincense, myrrh, nutmeg, lavender, lemon.

**ORANGE/SWEET:** anticoagulant, antidepressant, antiinflammatory, antiseptic, antispasmodic, bactericidal, carminative, cholagogue, digestive, diuretic, expectorant, fungicidal, sedative, stimulant, stomachic, tonic.
**Blends well with**-bergamot, black pepper, cinnamon, clary sage, clove, eucalyptus, frankincense, geranium, ginger, grapefruit, jasmine, juniper, lavender, lemon, marjoram, myrrh, neroli, nutmeg, patchouli, rose, sandalwood, ylang-ylang.

**OREGANO:** analgesic, anthelmintic, antibacterial, antifungal, antimicrobial, antiseptic, antispasmodic, carminative, cholagogue, diuretic, emmenagogue, expectorant, fungicidal, tonic.
**Blends well with**-bergamot, cedarwood, chamomile, citronella, cypress, eucalyptus, lavender, lemon, orange, pine, rosemary, tea tree, thyme.

**PALMAROSA:** antibacterial, antifungal, antiseptic, antiviral, cytophylactic, digestive, febrifuge, nervine, stimulant, tonic.
**Blends well with**-bergamot, cedarwood, chamomile, coriander, clary sage, clove, frankincense, geranium, ginger, grapefruit, juniper, lemon, lemongrass, mandarin, oakmoss, orange, patchouli, rose, rosemary, sandalwood, ylang-ylang.

**PALO SANTO:** antiinfectious, antitumor, antiviral, antiseptic, antiinflammatory, immunostimulant, sedative.
**Blends well with**-black pepper, cedarwood, clary sage, cypress, frankincense, lemon balm, rose, sandalwood.

**PARSLEY SEED:** antimicrobial, antiseptic, astringent, carminative, depurative, diuretic, emmenagogue, febrifuge, hypotensive, laxative, stimulant, stomachic, tonic.
**Blends well with**-black pepper, clary sage, ginger, neroli, rose, tea tree, ylang-ylang.

**PATCHOULI:** antibacterial, antidepressant, antiemetic, antiinflammatory, antiinflammatory, antimicrobial, antiphlogistic, antiseptic, antiviral, aphrodisiac, astringent, bactericidal, carminative, cicatrizant, cytophylactic, decongestant, diuretic, febrifuge, fungicidal, insecticide, laxative, nervine, sedative, stimulant, stomachic, tonic.

***Blends well with***-bergamot, black pepper, cedarwood, chamomile, cinnamon, clary sage, clove, frankincense, geranium, ginger, grapefruit, jasmine, lavender, lemongrass, neroli, orange, rose, sandalwood.

**PEPPERMINT:** analgesic, antibacterial, antifungal, antiinflammatory, antimicrobial, antiseptic, antispasmodic, astringent, carminative, cholagogue, decongestant, digestive, emmenagogue, expectorant, febrifuge, hepatic, insecticide, nervine, sedative, stimulant, stomachic, sudorific, vasoconstrictor, vermifuge.
***Blends well with*-**basil, black pepper, eucalyptus, geranium, grapefruit, juniper, lavender, lemon, marjoram, pine, rosemary, tea tree.

**PETITGRAIN:** antidepressant, antiseptic, antispasmodic, bactericidal, carminative, digestive, diuretic, emmenagogue, fungicidal, insecticide, nervine, sedative, stimulant, stomachic, tonic.
***Blends well with*-**bergamot, cedarwood, clary sage, clove, eucalyptus, frankincense, geranium, jasmine, juniper, lavender, lemon, marjoram, neroli, orange, tea, rose, rosemary, sandalwood, ylang-ylang.

**PIMENTO: (see allspice)** anesthetic, analgesic, antioxidant, antiseptic, relaxant, carminative, rubefacient, stimulant, tonic.

**PINE:** antimicrobial, antineuralgic, antirheumatic, antiseptic, antiviral, bactericidal, balsamic, cholagogue, diuretic, expectorant, hypertensive, insecticide, rubefacient, stimulant, tonic.
***Blends well with*-**bergamot, cedarwood, clary sage, cypress, eucalyptus, frankincense, grapefruit, juniper, lavender, lemon, marjoram, peppermint, rosemary, sage, sandalwood, tea tree, thyme.

# Oil Search R-Z

**RAVENSARA:** analgesic, antibacterial, antiinfectious, antimicrobial, antiseptic, antiviral, carminative, diuretic, expectorant, stimulant.
***Blends well with***-bergamot, black pepper, cedarwood, clary sage, cypress, eucalyptus, frankincense, geranium, ginger, grapefruit, lavender, lemon, marjoram, pine, rosemary, sandalwood, tea tree, thyme.

**ROSE:** analgesic, antibacterial, antidepressant, antifungal, antimicrobial, antiseptic, antispasmodic, antiviral, aphrodisiac, astringent, bactericidal, cholagogue, cicatrizant, depurative, disinfectant, diuretic, emmenagogue, hepatic, laxative, sedative, stomachic, tonic.
***Blends well with***-bergamot, chamomile, clary sage, fennel, geranium, ginger, helichrysum, jasmine, lavender, lemon, mandarin, neroli, patchouli, petitgrain, sandalwood, ylang-ylang, vetiver.

**ROSEMARY:** analgesic, antiarthritic, antibacterial, antidepressant, antioxidant, antirheumatic, antiseptic, antispasmodic, aphrodisiac, astringent, carminative, cephalic, cholagogue, decongestant, diaphoretic, digestive, diuretic, emmenagogue, expectorant, fungicidal, hepatic, hypertensive, nervine, rubefacient, stimulant, stomachic, sudorific, tonic, vermifuge, vulnerary.
***Blends well with***-basil, bergamot, black pepper, cedarwood, cinnamon, citronella, clary sage, eucalyptus, frankincense, geranium, grapefruit, lavender, lemon, mandarin, marjoram, oregano, peppermint, pine, tea tree, thyme.

**ROSEWOOD:** antidepressant, antiseptic, bactericidal, cephalic, cytophylactic, insecticide, stimulant.
***Blends well with***-bergamot, grapefruit, lemon, lime, neroli, lavender, jasmine, rose, orange.

**SAGE:** antibacterial, antiinflammatory, antimicrobial, antioxidant, antiseptic, antispasmodic, astringent, digestive, diuretic, emmenagogue, febrifuge, insecticide, laxative, stomachic, tonic.
***Blends well with***-citrus oils, hyssop, lavender, lemon, pine, rosemary, rosewood.

**SANDALWOOD:** antiinflammatory, antiphlogistic, antiseptic, antispasmodic, aphrodisiac, astringent, bactericidal, carminative, cicatrizant, decongestant, diuretic, emollient, expectorant, fungicidal, insecticide, sedative, tonic.
*Blends well with*-bergamot, black pepper, chamomile, clary sage, clove, geranium, grapefruit, frankincense, jasmine, lavender, lemon, myrrh, neroli, orange, palmarosa, patchouli, rose, vetiver, ylang-ylang.

**SPEARMINT:** analgesic, anesthetic, antibacterial, antiinflammatory, antiinflammatory, antiseptic, antispasmodic, astringent, carminative, cephalic, cholagogue, decongestant, digestive, diuretic, emmenagogue, expectorant, febrifuge, hepatic, insecticide, nervine, stimulant, stomachic, tonic.
*Blends well with*-basil, eucalyptus, jasmine, lavender, lemon, orange, peppermint, rosemary.

**SPIKENARD:** antibacterial, antibiotic, antifungal, antiinfectious, antiinflammatory, antiseptic, bactericidal, diuretic, fungicidal, laxative, sedative, tonic.
*Blends well with*-clary sage, clove, cypress, frankincense, geranium, lavender, lemon, neroli, patchouli, pine, rose.

**SPRUCE:** antibacterial, anticancer, antiinfectious, antiinflammatory, antimicrobial, antiseptic, antispasmodic, antiviral, astringent, diaphoretic, disinfectant, diuretic, expectorant, nervine, rubefacient, stimulant, tonic.
*Blends well with*-cedarwood, clary sage, lavender, pine, rosemary.

**ST. JOHN'S WORT:** analgesic, antibacterial, antidepressant, antiinflammatory, antimicrobial, antiseptic, antiviral, astringent, nervine, vulnerary.
*Blends well with*-helichrysum, lavender, wintergreen.

**TAGETES:** antispasmodic, bactericidal, carminative, diaphoretic, emmenagogue, fungicidal, stomachic.
*Blends well with*-bergamot, citrus oils, clary sage, jasmine, lavender, lemon.

**TANGERINE:** antimicrobial, antiseptic, antispasmodic, carminative, cytophylactic, depurative, digestive, diuretic, hypnotic, laxative, sedative, stimulant, stomachic, tonic.

***Blends well with**-basil, black pepper, chamomile, cinnamon, clary sage, clove, frankincense, geranium, grapefruit, jasmine, juniper, lemon, myrrh, neroli, nutmeg, patchouli, rose, sandalwood, ylang-ylang.

**TANSY:** analgesic, antibacterial, anticoagulant, antifungal, antiinfectious, antiinflammatory, antispasmodic, antiviral, insect-repellent, nervine, stimulant.
***Blends well with**-cedarwood, chamomile, copaiba, helichrysum, lavender, pine, ravensara, rosemary.

**TARRAGON:** antiseptic, antispasmodic, aperitive, carminative, digestive, diuretic, emmenagogue, hypnotic, stimulant, stomachic, vermifuge.
***Blends well with**-anise, basil, cistus, fennel, galbanum, lavender, oakmoss, lime, vanilla.

**TEA TREE/MALALEUCA:** analgesic, antibacterial, antifungal, antiinflammatory, antimicrobial, antiparasitic, antiseptic, antiviral, cicatrizant, decongestant, diaphoretic, expectorant, fungicidal, immunostimulant, insecticide, stimulant, sudorific, vulnerary.
***Blends well with**-bergamot, black pepper, chamomile, clary sage, clove, cypress, eucalyptus, geranium, juniper, lavender, lemon, nutmeg, oregano, peppermint, pine, ravensara, rosemary, thyme, ylang-ylang.

**THYME:** analgesic, anthelmintic, antibacterial, antifungal, antiinflammatory, antimicrobial, antioxidant, antirheumatic, antiseptic, antispasmodic, antiviral, bactericidal, carminative, cicatrizant, diuretic, emmenagogue, expectorant, insecticide, parasiticide, rubefacient, stimulant, tonic, vermifuge.
***Blends well with**-bergamot, clary sage, cypress, eucalyptus, geranium, grapefruit, lavender, lemon, lemon balm, marjoram, pine, rosemary, tea tree.

**TUMERIC:** analgesic, antiarthritic, antifungal, antiinflammatory, antioxidant, cholagogue, digestive, diuretic, insecticide, stimulant.
***Blends well with**-cistus, clary sage, ginger, ylang-ylang.

**VALERIAN:** antibacterial, antispasmodic, bactericidal, carminative, diuretic, hypnotic, hypotensive, sedative, stomachic.
***Blends well with**-cedarwood, lavender, mandarin, oakmoss, patchouli, petitgrain, pine, rosemary.

**VANILLA:** analgesic, antibacterial, anticonvulsant, antidepressant, anti-diuretic, antipyretic, antispasmodic, carminative, diuretic, febrifuge, hepatic, hypotensive, nervine, sedative, stomachic, tonic, vermifuge.
***Blends well with*-**benzoin, bergamot, frankincense, jasmine, lemon, mandarin, orange, patchouli, rose, sandalwood, vetiver, ylang-ylang.

**VETIVER:** analgesic, antibacterial, antifungal, antiinflammatory, antiinflammatory, antimicrobial, antioxidant, antiseptic, antispasmodic, depurative, emmenagogue, nervine, rubefacient, sedative, stimulant, tonic, vermifuge, vulnerary.
***Blends well with*-**bergamot, black pepper, cedarwood, clary sage, geranium, ginger, grapefruit, jasmine, lavender, lemon, lemongrass, mandarin, orange, patchouli, rose, sandalwood, ylang-ylang.

**WHITE FIR:** analgesic, antiarthritic, anticatarrhal, antioxidant, antiseptic, expectorant, stimulant.
***Blends well with*-**German male, cedarwood, cypress, frankincense, juniper, lavender, lemon, myrtle, pine, sandalwood, rosewood.

**WINTERGREEN:** analgesic, anticoagulant, antiinflammatory, antirheumatic, antiseptic, antispasmodic, disinfectant, vasodilator.
***Blends well with*-**oregano, peppermint, thyme, ylang-ylang.

**YARROW:** antiarthritic, antibacterial, antifungal, antiinflammatory, antipyretic, antirheumatic, antiseptic, antispasmodic, astringent, carminative, cicatrizant, diaphoretic, digestive, emmenagogue, expectorant, febrifuge, stimulant, stomachic, tonic, vulnerary.
***Blends well with*-**black pepper, bergamot, cedarwood, chamomile, clary sage, cypress, grapefruit, lavender, neroli, pine, vetiver, ylang-ylang.

**YLANG YLANG:** antibacterial, antidepressant, antifungal, antiinflammatory, antiinflammatory, antiseptic, antispasmodic, aphrodisiac, disinfectant, expectorant, hypotensive, nervine, sedative, vulnerary.
***Blends well with*-**bergamot, chamomile, clary sage, clove, eucalyptus, ginger, grapefruit, jasmine, ledum, mandarin, neroli, orange, patchouli, balsam, rose, rosewood, sandalwood.

# Property Search A-A

**ANALGESIC** (pain reliever) *allspice, anise seed, basil, bay laurel, bay West Indies, bergamot, birch, black pepper, blue tansy, cajeput, camphor, chamomile-German, chamomile-Roman, cilantro, cinnamon, citronella, clove, copaiba, coriander, dorado azil, elemi, eucalyptus, fennel, fir needle, frankincense, galbanum, geranium, ginger, ho wood, jasmine, juniper berry, lavandin, lavender, lemongrass, mace, manuka, marjoram, niaouli, nutmeg, oregano, peppermint, pimento, ravensara, rose, rosemary, spearmint, St. John's wort, tansy, tea tree/malaleuca, thyme, tumeric, vanilla, vetiver, white fir, wintergreen*

**ANAPHRODISIAC** (decreases libido/sex drive) *marjoram*

**ANESTHETIC** (causes reversible loss of sensation) *allspice, bay laurel, blue tansy, catnip, cornmint, fennel, manuka, pimento, spearmint*

**ANTHELMINTIC see also "antiparasitic"** (causes expelling of parasites) *bergamot, carrot seed, oregano, thyme*

**ANTIAGING** (works against normal aging) *clove*

**ANTIARTHRITIC see also "antiinflammatory"** (prevents or relieves arthritic symptoms) *cassia, rosemary, tumeric, white fir, yarrow*

**ANTIBACTERIAL** (destroys or prevents bacterial growth) *allspice, angelica, basil, bay laurel, bergamot, black pepper, blue tansy, cajeput, cardamom, chamomile-Roman, cinnamon, citronella, clary sage, clove, copaiba, cypress, eucalyptus, geranium, ginger, grapefruit, helichrysum, hinoki, hyssop, Idaho blue spruce, lavender, ledum, lemon, lemon balm (melissa), lime, litsea cubeba, manuka, mountain savory, myrtle, neroli, oregano, palmarosa, patchouli, peppermint, ravensara, rose, rosemary, sage, spearmint, spikenard, spruce, St. John's wort, tansy, tea tree/malaleuca, thyme, valerian, vanilla, vetiver, yarrow, ylang ylang*

**ANTIBIOTIC see "antibacterial"** (treats bacterial infections) *litsea cubeba, spikenard*

**ANTICANCER** (fights against cancer) *dorado azil, Idaho blue spruce, ledum, spruce*

**ANTICATARRHAL see "mucolytic"** (removes excess mucous from body) *frankincense, myrrh, myrtle, niaouli, white fir*

**ANTICOAGULANT** (blood thinner) *balsam fir, cinnamon, clove, ginger, helichrysum, orange/sweet, tansy, wintergreen*

**ANTICONVULSANT** (prevents or reduces severity/frequency of seizures) *bay laurel, bay West Indies, vanilla*

**ANTIDEPRESSANT** (combats depressive disorders, anxiety/depression etc.) *basil, benzoin, bergamot, cassia, clary sage, frankincense, geranium, grapefruit, jasmine, lavandin, lavender, lemongrass, melissa, neroli, orange/bitter, orange/sweet, patchouli, petitgrain, rose, rosemary, rosewood, St. John's wort, vanilla, ylang ylang, antibacterial*

**ANTIDIABETIC** (assists in control of glucose/sugar levels) *geranium*

**ANTIDIARRHEAL** (assists in combating diarrhea) *cassia*

**ANTIEMETIC** (fights vomiting and nausea) *cassia, patchouli, peppermint, spearmint, ginger,*

**ANTIFUNGAL** (an agent to prevent or treat fungal infections) *allspice, angelica, bay laurel, black pepper, cedarwood, cinnamon, citronella, clove, dorado azil, Douglas fir, eucalyptus, frankincense, hinoki, lemon, lemongrass, manuka, mountain savory, myrrh, oregano, palmarosa, peppermint, rose, spikenard, tansy, tea tree/malaleuca, thyme, tumeric, vetiver, yarrow, ylang ylang*

**ANTIHISTAMINE** (an agent to prevent or reduce allergic reaction) *blue tansy, lemon balm (melissa)*

**ANTIINFECTIOUS** (fights or prevents infection) *dorado azil, hinoki, Idaho blue spruce, litsea cubeba, mountain savory, palo santo, ravensara, spikenard, spruce, tansy*

**ANTIINFLAMMATORY** (prevents or reduces tissue inflammation) *balsam fir, basil, benzoin, blue cypress, blue tansy, camphor, catnip,* *chamomile-German, chamomile-Roman, cilantro, cinnamon, clove, copaiba, cypress, dorado azil, frankincense, galbanum, geranium, ginger, goldenrod, helichrysum, Idaho blue spruce, jasmine, lavender, ledum, lemon, lemon balm (melissa), lemongrass, litsea cubeba, manuka, mountain savory, myrrh, neroli, nutmeg, orange/bitter, palo santo, patchouli, peppermint, sandalwood, spearmint, spikenard, spruce, St. John's wort, tansy, vetiver, yarrow, ylang ylang*

**ANTI-ITCH see also "antihistamine"** (helps relieve itching) *blue tansy*

**ANTIMICROBIAL** (an agent that kills or prohibits growth of certain microorganisms) *bay laurel, benzoin, black pepper, cajeput, cassia, chamomile-Roman, cinnamon, cistus, clove, cornmint, dorado azil, fennel, galbanum, helichrysum, hinoki, hops, juniper berry, lavender, lemon, lemongrass, lovage leaf, manuka, myrrh, oregano, parsley seed, patchouli, peppermint, pine, ravensara, rose, sage, spruce, St. John's wort, tangerine, tea tree/malaleuca, thyme, vetiver*

**ANTINEURALGIC see "antiinflammatory"** (relief of nerve-type pain) *bay West Indies, cajeput, chamomile-Roman, eucalyptus, pine*

**ANTIOXIDANT** (an agent that helps to prevent cell damage from oxidation) *allspice, cilantro, clove, dorado azil, frankincense, ginger, helichrysum, lemongrass, mace, marjoram, nutmeg, pimento, rosemary, sage, thyme, tumeric, vetiver, white fir*

**ANTIPARASITIC see "anthelmintic"** (removes or prevents parasites) *lemongrass, mountain savory, tea tree/malaleuca*

**ANTIPHLOGISTIC** (fights fever or inflammation) *chamomile-German, chamomile-Roman, clary sage, patchouli, sandalwood*

**ANTIPUTREFACTIVE** (preserving) *juniper berry*

**ANTIPYRETIC see "febrifuge"** (reduces fever) *vanilla, yarrow*

**ANTIRHEUMATIC** (relieves or prevents rheumatism) *bay laurel, cassia, catnip, celery seed, eucalyptus, hyssop, juniper berry, lavender, lemon, niaouli, nutmeg, pine, rosemary, thyme, wintergreen, yarrow*

**ANTISEBORRHEIC** (prevents or relieves seborrhea) *cedarwood*

**ANTISEPTIC** (discourages the growth of microorganisms) *allspice, amyris, angelica, anise seed, balsam fir, basil, bay laurel, bay West Indies, benzoin, bergamot, birch, black pepper, cajeput, camphor, cardamom, carrot seed, cedarwood, celery seed, chamomile-Roman, cinnamon, cistus, citronella, clary sage, clove, copaiba, cornmint, cypress, davana, Douglas fir, elemi, eucalyptus, fennel, fir needle, frankincense, galbanum, geranium, ginger, grapefruit, helichrysum, hinoki, ho wood, hops, hyssop, Idaho blue spruce, jasmine, juniper berry, lavandin, lavender, lemon, lemon balm (melissa), lemongrass, lime, litsea cubeba, lovage leaf, mandarin, manuka, marjoram, myrrh, myrtle, neroli, niaouli, nutmeg, oak moss, orange/bitter, orange/sweet, oregano, palmarosa, palo santo, parsley seed, patchouli, peppermint, petitgrain, pimento, pine, ravensara, rose, rosemary, rosewood, sage, sandalwood, spearmint, spikenard, spruce, St. John's wort, tangerine, tarragon, tea tree/malaleuca, thyme, vetiver, white fir, wintergreen, yarrow, ylang ylang*

**ANTISPASMODIC see "muscle relaxant"** (an agent that suppresses muscle spasm) *angelica, anise seed, basil, bergamot, black pepper, cajeput, camphor, cardamom, catnip, cedarwood, celery seed, chamomile-German, chamomile-Roman, cilantro, cinnamon, citronella, clary sage, clove, coriander, cornmint, cypress, dill seed, eucalyptus, fennel, galbanum, ginger, helichrysum, hops, hyssop, Idaho blue spruce, jasmine, juniper berry, lavender, lemon, lemon balm (melissa), lime, lovage leaf, mace, mandarin, marjoram, melissa, myrrh, neroli, niaouli, nutmeg, orange/bitter, orange/sweet, oregano, peppermint, petitgrain, rose, rosemary, sage, sandalwood, spearmint, spruce, tagetes, tangerine, tansy, tarragon, thyme, valerian, vanilla, vetiver, wintergreen, yarrow, ylang ylang*

**ANTITUMOR** (prevents or reduces tumors) *palo santo*

**ANTITUSSIVE** (prevents or relieves cough) *douglas fir, fir needle, frankincense, eucalyptus*

**ANTIVIRAL** (prevents or treats viral infections) *allspice, bergamot, blue cypress, camphor, cassia, clove, davana, elemi, eucalyptus, hinoki, hyssop, Idaho blue spruce, lavender, ledum, lemon balm (melissa), lemongrass, lime, mandarin, manuka, marjoram, melissa, mountain savory, myrrh, palmarosa, palo santo, patchouli, pine, ravensara, rose, spruce, St. John's wort, tansy, tea tree/malaleuca, thyme*

**APERITIVE** (stimulates appetite) *anise seed, bay laurel, black pepper, cilantro, fennel, ginger, lime, nutmeg, tarragon*

**APHRODISIAC** (increases/stimulates libido/sex drive) *allspice, cardamom, clary sage, coriander, davana, ginger, jasmine, mace, marjoram, neroli, nutmeg, patchouli, rose, rosemary, sandalwood, ylang ylang*

**ASTRINGENT** (contracting, constrictive, styptic, cleaning) *balsam fir, bay West Indies, benzoin, bergamot, cassia, catnip, cedarwood, cinnamon, cistus, citronella, clary sage, cypress, eucalyptus, fir needle, frankincense, geranium, grapefruit, helichrysum, hinoki, hops, hyssop, juniper berry, lemon, lemongrass, lime, myrrh, myrtle, orange/bitter, parsley seed, patchouli, peppermint, rose, rosemary, sage, sandalwood, spearmint, spruce, St. John's wort, yarrow*

# Property Search B-E

**BACTERICIDAL** (an agent that kills bacteria) *camphor, black pepper, blue cypress, blue tansy, cajeput, camphor, cardamom, carrot seed, cassia, catnip, cedarwood, celery seed, chamomile-German, chamomile-Roman, cilantro, coriander, dill seed, hops, lavender, lemon balm (melissa), lemongrass, lime, marjoram, melissa, myrtle, lovage leaf, mace, mandarin, manuka, marjoram, melaleuca/tea tree, melissa, mountain savory, myrrh, myrtle, neroli, niaouli, orange/bitter, orange/sweet, nutmeg, oak moss, oregano, palmarosa, palo santo, parsley seed, patchouli, peppermint, petitgrain, pimento, pine, rose, rosewood, sandalwood, ravensara, rosemary, sage, sandalwood, spearmint, spikenard, tagetes, thyme, valerian*

**BALSAMIC** (containing balsam) *amyris, galbanum, pine*

**CALMATIVE** (has a calming effect) *douglas fir*

**CARMINATIVE** (assists in preventing or expelling intestinal gas/flatulence) *allspice, angelica, anise seed, basil, bay laurel, benzoin, bergamot, black pepper, cajeput, cardamom, carrot seed, cassia, catnip, celery seed, black pepper, blue cypress, blue tansy, cajeput, camphor, cardamom, carrot seed, cassia, catnip, cedarwood, celery seed, chamomile-German, chamomile-Roman, cinnamon, clary sage, clove, coriander, cornmint, ginger, hops, hyssop, geranium, ginger, goldenrod, grapefruit, helichrysum, hinoki, ho wood, hops, hyssop, Idaho blue spruce, juniper berry, lavender, lemon, lemon balm (melissa), lemongrass, lime, jasmine, lavandin, ledum, litsea cubeba, lovage leaf, mace, mandarin, marjoram, melissa, myrrh, neroli, nutmeg, orange/bitter, orange/sweet, oregano, parsley seed, patchouli, peppermint, nutmeg, oak moss, palmarosa, palo santo, petitgrain, pimento, ravensara, rosemary, sandalwood, spearmint, tagetes, tangerine, tarragon, thyme, valerian, spikenard, spruce, St. John's wort, tansy, tea tree/malaleuca, thyme, tumeric, valerian, vanilla, yarrow*

**CEPHALIC** (relating to the head) basil, *cardamom, ginger, hyssop, marjoram, rosemary, rosewood, spearmint*

**CHOLAGOGUE** (stimulates gallbladder to promote bile flow) *angelica, chamomile-Roman, ginger, helichrysum, lavender, mace, mandarin, nutmeg, orange/sweet, oregano, peppermint, pine, rose, rosemary, spearmint, tumeric*

**CICATRIZANT** (promotes healing thru scar tissue formation) *bergamot, black pepper, blue cypress, blue tansy, cajeput, camphor, cardamom, carrot seed, cassia, catnip, cedarwood, celery seed, chamomile-German, elemi, eucalyptus, frankincense, geranium, helichrysum, hyssop, lavandin, lavender, lemon, myrrh, neroli, lovage leaf, mace, mandarin, manuka, marjoram, melaleuca/tea tree, melissa, mountain savory, myrrh, myrtle, neroli, niaouli, patchouli, rose, sandalwood, tea tree/malaleuca, thyme, yarrow*

**CIRCULATORY** (assists the circulatory system) *cassia, cedarwood*

**COOLING** (produces a cooling effect on the body) *bergamot, peppermint*

**CYTOPHYLACTIC** (promotes new cell growth) *carrot seed, frankincense, geranium, lavender, palmarosa, patchouli, rosewood, tangerine*

**DECONGESTANT** (relieves congestion in the nasal/upper airway region) *amyris, cajeput, camphor, eucalyptus, hinoki, lavender, lovage leaf, mace, mandarin, manuka, marjoram, melaleuca/tea tree, melissa, mountain savory, myrrh, myrtle, neroli, niaouli, patchouli, peppermint, rosemary, sandalwood, spearmint, tea tree/malaleuca*

**DEMULCENT** (relieves irritation of the oral mucous membranes) *oak moss*

**DEPURATIVE** (having purifying and detoxifying effects) *angelica, birch, carrot seed, cilantro, cardamom coriander, eucalyptus, fennel, grapefruit, juniper berry, lemon, mandarin, parsley seed, rose, tangerine, vetiver*

**DETOXICANT see also "depurative"** (detoxifies) *juniper berry*

**DIAPHORETIC see "sudorific"** (makes you sweat) *angelica, bay laurel, black pepper, cajeput, catnip, cedarwood, citronella, ginger, lemon, lemon balm (melissa), jasmine, juniper berry, lavandin, lavender, ledum, lemon, lemon balm (melissa), lemongrass, lime, litsea* *cubeba, lovage leaf, marjoram, melissa, lovage leaf, mace, mandarin, manuka, melaleuca/tea tree, mountain savory, myrrh, myrtle, neroli, niaouli, rosemary, spruce, tagetes, tea tree/malaleuca, yarrow*

**DIGESTIVE see "stomachic"** (assists the GI tract) *angelica, anise seed, basil, bergamot, black pepper, cardamom, celery seed, black pepper, blue cypress, blue tansy, cajeput, camphor, cardamom, carrot seed, cassia, catnip, cedarwood, celery seed, chamomile-German, chamomile-Roman, cilantro, cardamom cinnamon, clary sage, coriander, cornmint, ginger, grapefruit, hyssop, juniper berry, lemon, lemon balm (melissa), lemongrass, litsea cubeba, jasmine, juniper berry, lavandin, lavender, ledum, lovage leaf, mandarin, marjoram, myrrh, neroli, nutmeg, orange/bitter, orange/sweet, palmarosa, peppermint, nutmeg, oak moss, oregano, palo santo, parsley seed, patchouli, petitgrain, rosemary, sage, spearmint, tangerine, tarragon, tumeric, yarrow*

**DISINFECTANT** (destroys bacteria) *birch, copaiba, davana, Douglas fir, grapefruit, Idaho blue spruce, lime, rose, spruce, wintergreen, ylang ylang*

**DIURETIC** (increases production of urine) *angelica, anise seed, bay laurel, benzoin, bergamot, birch, black pepper, camphor, cardamom, carrot seed, cedarwood, celery seed, citronella, copaiba, cypress, eucalyptus, fennel, frankincense, galbanum, geranium, ginger, goldenrod, grapefruit, helichrysum, hops, hyssop, juniper berry, lavender, ledum, lemon, jasmine, juniper berry, lavandin, lemon balm (melissa), lemongrass, lime, litsea cubeba, lovage leaf, mandarin, marjoram, orange/sweet, oregano, parsley seed, patchouli, nutmeg, oak moss, palo santo, peppermint, petitgrain, pine, ravensara, rose, rosemary, sage, sandalwood, spearmint, pimento, rosewood, spikenard, spruce, tangerine, tarragon, St. John's wort, tagetes, tansy, tea tree/malaleuca, thyme, tumeric, valerian, vanilla*

**EMMENAGOGUE** (promotes blood flow to pelvis/uterus) *angelica, anise seed, basil, carrot seed, cassia, cedarwood, celery seed, chamomile-German, chamomile-Roman, cistus, citronella, clary sage, cypress, davana, dill seed, fennel, frankincense, galbanum, geranium, hyssop, geranium, ginger, goldenrod, grapefruit, helichrysum, hinoki, ho wood, hops, Idaho blue spruce, juniper berry, lemon balm (melissa), jasmine, juniper berry, lavandin, lavender, ledum, lemon, lemon balm (melissa), lemongrass, lime, litsea cubeba, lovage leaf, marjoram, melissa, myrrh, nutmeg, oregano, oak moss, orange/bitter,* orange/sweet, palmarosa, palo santo, parsley seed, patchouli, peppermint, petitgrain, rose, rosemary, sage, spearmint, tagetes, tarragon, thyme, vetiver, yarrow

**EMOLLIENT see also "skin"** (softens and soothes skin) *amyris, sandalwood*

**EXPECTORANT** (assists in breaking and bringing up lung/tracheal mucous) *angelica, anise seed, balsam fir, basil, bay laurel, bay West Indies, benzoin, bergamot, cajeput, camphor, cedarwood, cinnamon, cistus, clove, copaiba, cornmint, ginger, helichrysum, hyssop, Idaho blue spruce, geranium, ginger, goldenrod, grapefruit, hinoki, ho wood, hops, hyssop, lavandin, jasmine, juniper berry, lavender, ledum, lemon, lemon balm (melissa), lemongrass, lime, litsea cubeba, lovage leaf, manuka, marjoram, myrrh, myrtle, mace, mandarin, manuka, marjoram, melaleuca/tea tree, melissa, mountain savory, neroli, niaouli, oak moss, orange/sweet, oregano, peppermint, pine, ravensara, rosemary, sandalwood, spearmint, spruce, tea tree/malaleuca, thyme, white fir, yarrow, ylang ylang*

# Property Search F-M

**FEBRIFUGE see "antipyretic"** (reduces fever) *angelica, basil, bergamot, birch, black pepper, cajeput, cassia, chamomile-German, chamomile-Roman, citronella, cypress, eucalyptus, ginger, hyssop, lemon balm (melissa), lemongrass, lime, jasmine, juniper berry, lavandin, lavender, ledum, lemon, lemongrass, litsea cubeba, lovage leaf, melissa, mace, mandarin, manuka, marjoram, melaleuca/tea tree, melissa, mountain savory, myrrh, myrtle, neroli, niaouli, palmarosa, parsley seed, patchouli, peppermint, sage, spearmint, spruce, St. John's wort, tagetes, tangerine, tansy, tarragon, tea tree/malaleuca, thyme, tumeric, valerian, vanilla, yarrow*

**FIBROMYALGIA** (chronic body wide pain in muscles and connective tissues) *helichrysum, lemon, tea tree/malaleuca, oregano, lavender, basil, marjoram, peppermint, thyme, orange*

**FUNGICIDAL** (kills or prohibits fungus growth) *cedarwood, chamomile-German, cilantro, cardamom citronella, coriander, elemi, lemongrass, marjoram, myrrh, neroli, orange/bitter, orange/sweet, oregano, nutmeg, oak moss, palo santo, parsley seed, patchouli, peppermint, petitgrain, sandalwood, petitgrain, pimento, pine, ravensara, rose, rosemary, rosewood, sage, sandalwood, spearmint, spikenard, tagetes, tea tree/malaleuca*

**GALACTAGOGUE** (promotes female lactation/breast milk) *cassia, celery seed, fennel, geranium, ginger, goldenrod, grapefruit, helichrysum, hinoki, ho wood, hops, hyssop, Idaho blue spruce*

**HEMOSTATIC** (styptic, stops bleeding) *cypress, geranium, lime*

**HEPATIC** (works on the liver, promotes health) *carrot seed, celery seed, chamomile-German, chamomile-Roman, cypress, geranium, helichrysum, peppermint, rose, spearmint, spruce, St. John's wort, tagetes, tangerine, tansy, tarragon, tea tree/malaleuca, thyme, tumeric, valerian, vanilla*

**HYPERTENSIVE** (works on blood pressure) *goldenrod, hyssop, pine*

**HYPNOTIC** (assists in hypnosis, calming, soothing) *mandarin, tangerine, tarragon, valerian*

**HYPOTENSIVE** (lowers blood pressure) *blue tansy, clary sage, dill seed, galbanum, lemon, marjoram, melissa, parsley seed, valerian, spruce, St. John's wort, tagetes, tangerine, tansy, tarragon, tea tree/malaleuca, thyme, tumeric, vanilla, ylang ylang*

**IMMUNOSTIMULANT** (stimulates the immune system) *Idaho blue spruce, manuka, mountain savory, palo santo, tea tree/malaleuca*

**INSECTICIDE** (kills or prevents insect growth) *birch, cajeput, catnip, cedarwood, clove, cypress, dorado azil, eucalyptus, geranium, hinoki, lemon, lemongrass, lime, litsea cubeba, manuka, lovage leaf, mace, mandarin, manuka, marjoram, melaleuca/tea tree, melissa, mountain savory, myrrh, peppermint, petitgrain, pine, rosewood, sage, sandalwood, tea tree/malaleuca, thyme, tumeric*

**INSECT-REPELLENT** *blue cypress, cajeput, catnip, cedarwood, citronella, clove, eucalyptus, lemongrass, rosemary, tea tree, tansy, lavender, peppermint*

**LAXATIVE** (encourages peristalsis, bowel movement) *bergamot, black pepper, cardamom, fennel, ginger, lemon, mace, mandarin, marjoram, nutmeg, parsley seed, rose, sage, petitgrain, pimento, pine, ravensara, rosemary, rosewood, sandalwood, spearmint, spikenard, tangerine*

**LIPOLYTIC** (breaks down fats into fatty acids) *coriander*

**LIVER** (promotes liver health) *goldenrod, lemon, peppermint, grapefruit, myrrh, clove, geranium, rosemary*

**MUCOLYTIC see "anticatarrhal"** (loosens/clears mucous from the airway) *helichrysum, hinoki*

**MUSCLE RELAXANT see "antispasmodic"** *amyris*

# Property Search N-Z

**NAUSEA/VOMITING** see "antiemetic"

**NERVINE** (having a beneficial effect on the nervous system) *angelica, basil, blue tansy, catnip, celery seed, chamomile-German, chamomile-Roman, clary sage, davana, Douglas fir, helichrysum, hops, hyssop, lavandin, ledine, lemon balm (melissa), lemongrass, manuka, marjoram, melissa, neroli, palmarosa, peppermint, petitgrain, spruce, St. John's wort, tansy, tagetes, tangerine, tarragon, tea tree/malaleuca, thyme, tumeric, valerian, vanilla, vetiver, ylang ylang*

**PARASITICIDE** (kills parasites) *thyme*

**RELAXANT** (an agent that relaxes) *amyris, blue tansy, clary sage, hinoki, geranium, ginger, goldenrod, grapefruit, helichrysum, ho wood, hops, hyssop, Idaho blue spruce, juniper berry, marjoram, pimento*

**RUBEFACIENT** (causes redness of the skin, increased blood capillary flow) *allspice, bergamot, black pepper, camphor, eucalyptus, fir needle, frankincense, geranium, ginger, juniper berry, lemon, pimento, pine, spruce, vetiver*

**SEDATIVE** (induces a sedating effect) *amyris, balsam fir, bay laurel, benzoin, bergamot, catnip, cedarwood, celery seed, chamomile-Roman, citronella, clary sage, cypress, davana, frankincense, geranium, ho wood, hops, hyssop, geranium, ginger, goldenrod, grapefruit, helichrysum, hinoki, ho wood, hops, hyssop, Idaho blue spruce, juniper berry, lemon balm (melissa), lemongrass, litsea cubeba, mandarin, manuka, marjoram, melissa, myrrh, myrtle, neroli, orange/bitter, orange/sweet, palo santo, peppermint, petitgrain, sandalwood, pimento, pine, ravensara, rose, rosemary, rosewood, sage, sandalwood, spearmint, spikenard, tangerine, valerian, spruce, St. John's wort, tagetes, tangerine, tansy, tarragon, tea tree/malaleuca, thyme, tumeric, valerian, vanilla, vetiver, ylang ylang*

**SPLENIC** (promotes spleen health) *fennel*

**STIMULANT** (stimulates the mind/body) *allspice, angelica, anise seed, basil, bay West Indies, bergamot, black pepper, blue cypress,* cajeput, camphor, cardamom, carrot seed, cassia, cilantro, cardamom cinnamon, citronella, clove, copaiba, coriander, cornmint, geranium, ginger, goldenrod, grapefruit, helichrysum, hyssop, Idaho blue spruce, juniper berry, ledum, lemongrass, litsea cubeba, jasmine, juniper berry, lavandin, lavender, lemon, lemon balm (melissa), lime, litsea cubeba, lovage leaf, mace, mandarin, manuka, mountain savory, marjoram, melaleuca/tea tree, melissa, myrrh, myrtle, neroli, niaouli, nutmeg, orange/bitter, orange/sweet, palmarosa, palo santo, parsley seed, petitgrain, pimento, pine, ravensara, rosewood, spruce, tangerine, tansy, tarragon, tea tree/malaleuca, tumeric, vetiver, white fir, yarrow

**STOMACHIC see "digestive"** (stomach toning, increased appetite) angelica, anise seed, basil, bergamot, black pepper, cardamom, celery seed, dill seed, Douglas fir, elemi, fennel, juniper berry, litsea cubeba, jasmine, juniper berry, lavandin, lavender, ledum, lemon, lemon balm (melissa), lemongrass, lime, litsea cubeba, lovage leaf, marjoram, melissa, myrrh, orange/bitter, orange/sweet, parsley seed, tagetes, tangerine, tarragon, valerian, spruce, St. John's wort, tansy, tea tree/malaleuca, thyme, tumeric, valerian, vanilla, yarrow

**STYPTIC** (stops bleeding) cypress, geranium, lime

**SUDORIFIC see "diaphoretic"** (causes sweating) basil, cajeput, camphor, chamomile-German, cypress, hyssop, juniper berry, melissa, tea tree/malaleuca

**TONIC** (health and well being restoration) angelica, balsam fir, basil, bay West Indies, bergamot, birch, black pepper, cajeput, cardamom, carrot seed, catnip, cedarwood, celery seed, cypress, Douglas fir, elemi, fennel, fir needle, frankincense, galbanum, geranium, ginger, goldenrod, grapefruit, helichrysum, hinoki, ho wood, hops, hyssop, Idaho blue spruce, juniper berry, ledum, lemon balm (melissa), lemongrass, lime, mace, mandarin, marjoram, melissa, myrrh, myrtle, neroli, nutmeg, orange/bitter, orange/sweet, oregano, palmarosa, parsley seed, petitgrain, pimento, pine, ravensara, rose, rosemary, rosewood, sage, sandalwood, spearmint, spikenard, spruce, tangerine, spruce, St. John's wort, tagetes, tansy, tarragon, tea tree/malaleuca, thyme, tumeric, valerian, vanilla, vetiver, yarrow

**UTERINE** (works to improve uterine function) geranium, ginger, goldenrod, grapefruit, helichrysum, hinoki, ho wood, hops, hyssop, Idaho blue spruce, myrrh

**VASOCONSTRICTOR** (constricts blood vessels) *cypress, peppermint*

**VASODILATOR** (dilates blood vessels) *black pepper, Douglas fir, wintergreen*

**VERMIFUGE** (destroys or expels parasites) *cajeput, camphor, carrot seed, chamomile-German, cinnamon, eucalyptus, fennel, hyssop, lemon balm (melissa), lovage leaf, mace, mandarin, manuka, marjoram, melaleuca/tea tree, melissa, mountain savory, myrrh, myrtle, neroli, niaouli, spruce, St. John's wort, tagetes, tangerine, tansy, tarragon, tea tree/malaleuca, thyme, tumeric, valerian, vanilla, vetiver*

**VULNERARY** (promotes wound healing) *benzoin, cajeput, camphor, chamomile-German, clary sage, davana, lavandin, litsea cubeba, manuka, lovage leaf, mace, mandarin, marjoram, melaleuca/tea tree, melissa, mountain savory, myrrh, myrtle, neroli, niaouli, St. John's wort, tea tree/malaleuca, vetiver, ylang ylang*

**WARMING** (warm to the body) *benzoin, birch, clary sage*

# Applying/Using Essential Oils

We use EOs by applying them to the *skin*, *inhaling* them (aromatherapy), or *ingesting* them. In each of these three avenues there are different application methods available. Most oils can be administered in any of these ways, but some ways are better than others for each oil and desired effect. Ingesting, especially, should be with care and knowledge. The vast majority of time you are better off not ingesting them (that's my opinion as there is usually no need).

Our bodies are amazing. Our skin is the largest organ of our body. The average adult has over 22 square feet of skin, over 8 pounds. Oils can be absorbed through the skin. That is why most EO experts advise against internal ingestion of oils. We don't have to swallow the oil for it to enter our bloodstream. Many biological weapons can kill you just from having your skin exposed to them.

Similarly, our lungs and oral mucosa readily **absorb oils directly** into our bloodstream. Thus the buccal/sublingual methods and aromatherapy work very well to get some of these oils into our blood and tissues for use.

Always skin patch test any oil you are using for the first time, regardless of the application method.

**INHALING** can be done through spraying, dry evaporation, diffuser/vaporizer devices or by steam.

To **spray** you can simply add some drops of your EO to a spray bottle with water in it, shake and spray into an open room, on your skin or wherever. This is one of the first things you might want to try. It can really change the atmosphere and mood in a room. It can also be used to disinfect things, disinfect the air and to help with bad odors etc. Always remember to shake the bottle before spraying. Oil travels quickly to the top of the water in the bottle. It will also want to cling to the sides of the bottle.

**Dry evaporation** is another great way to use EOs. You can simply place a few drops on a cotton ball, soft tissue or other throw-away material and inhale/smell directly or leave it somewhere close to you. You can be creative. You can make wonderful car fresheners. I often do this in my office while I'm working at the computer. It ALWAYS gives me a lift.

**Steam inhalation** can be accomplished by putting 1-2 drops of EO into steaming water. These oils vaporize quicker than the water so it can be very potent quickly. You let the vapors diffuse throughout the room and breathe in the vapors. It is easy, quick and effective, but be careful. **KNOW** the oil you are using.

**Diffusers and vaporizers** are devices that diffuse the oil into the surrounding air. They come in all kinds of shapes, styles and prices. Their job is to diffuse the oils into the air. Some diffusers use dry heat and some use steam. They are widely available at a wide range of prices.

**APPLICATION TO/THROUGH THE SKIN** can be accomplished a myriad of ways. Always remember, dilution with a carrier oil/medium is warranted most of the time. Carrier oils can be obtained through health food stores, the grocery store and usually wherever you purchase your EOs.

The most common **carrier oils** are olive oil, coconut oil and jojoba. Other carrier oils might include apricot kernel, almond, grapeseed, avocado, wheat germ or evening primrose.

**Massaging** generally works well at about 1% to 3% oil to the carrier. 1% equates to about 1 drop of EO in a teaspoon of carrier oil, 5 drops per teaspoon is about 5%. You use it as you would any massage oil. Massaging/rubbing the oil mixture directly over the affected part of the body is oftentimes one of the best methods for rapid absorption where it is needed.

You can pour about a teaspoon of carrier oil into our cupped hands; add a drop or two of oil and then use this as massage oil to the desired area.

The **bathtub** is a great place to add a little oil while you're soaking. Sometimes the benefits of this can be marvelous. It can do wonders to reduce stress, anxiety, muscle aches and pains, aid in sleeping, reduce restlessness, help to ease PMS symptoms and to soothe hemorrhoids. This can even help to ease ailments of the internal organs, such as the bladder, liver or kidneys. You can add anywhere from 1-9 drops of oil to a teaspoon of carrier and dump it into the already ran bathwater. Footbaths are great also.

You can add EOs to **compresses** for application to the skin. A compress is usually some type of cloth or material soaked in warm/hot or cold water, depending on the desired effect. The compress is placed and held against the skin.

Cold compresses can be applied to treat things like swollen joints, localized swelling, sprains, soft tissue injuries, bruises, headaches, insect bites and some skin infections. In short, anywhere you want inflammation and swelling to decrease.

Warm/hot compresses are usually used on things like stiff joints and muscle aches and pains. Generally, you should not use heat where there is swelling, at least until after you have applied a cold compress first.

I have also seen some serious burns, especially in the elderly or diabetics, from hot compresses left on too long. Most practitioners consider 20 minutes to be the maximum amount of time to apply a compress.

Cold compresses are often applied first to reduce swelling/inflammation. Then warm/hot compresses are applied to increase blood flow to the area after that. This is a fairly common practice in physical therapy and for sporting injuries.

Finally, some oils can be **ingested internally**. You generally want to know your oil well and make sure it is safe before ingesting. Some oils can be toxic or poisonous when taken internally. Some people say never ingest any EOs, which is ridiculous. All kinds of food you buy at the grocery store contain EOs and/or their components. A few drops of citrus oils can be added to a glass of water, stirred and drank.

Caution and a little research is the key. "First do no harm" should be a phrase we all keep in mind when it comes to these oils and our health in general.

# Blending Essential Oils

Synergy plays a major role in mixing and blending oils. Synergy is necessary for life. It is working everywhere around us all the time. In synergy, 1 + 1 can = 1000. Synergy is the creation of a whole that is greater than the sum of its parts.

Some oils can be mixed together with really nice results. There is a real art and science to mixing oils.

There are therapeutic blends and there are aromatic blends. Some people use oil vibration frequency to determine blending. There are many different types of methods used to determine blending.

Most of the time, aromatic blending will be seeking blends that smell really well together. Therapeutic blends on the other hand are seeking more of the medicinal effects versus pleasantness.

The groupings in this book should be of assistance to you when determining a blend of oils.

# References

EverythingEssential-Everything about essential oils

Jo's Health Corner-Blog

"Essential Oils for Beginners" by Julia Grady

"Essential Oils: Essential Oils For Beginners" Brene Farm

"Essential Oils 911 Ailments" by Kellie Christensen

"1001 Ways to Use Essential Oils" by Beth Jones

Young Living Essential Oils

Natural News

doTERRA

Wikipedia

If you find this book helpful, please leave a QUICK REVIEW on Amazon. That would be greatly appreciated. You can also see my OTHER BOOKS on EOs there as well. You can visit my website at chasharrison.com to sign up for free offers on eBooks, audio books and print offers.

Thank you for using this book.

Chas R. Harrison

# NOTES

# NOTES

# NOTES

Made in the USA
Middletown, DE
31 March 2017